The Food Combining
2-Day Detox

Kathryn Marsden

The Food Combining
2-Day Detox

PAN BOOKS

First published 1998 by Macmillan

an imprint of Macmillan Publishers Ltd
25 Eccleston Place, London SW1W 9NF
and Basingstoke

Associated companies throughout the world

ISBN 0 330 35483 3

Copyright © Kathryn Marsden 1998

The right of Kathryn Marsden to be identified as the
author of this work has been asserted by her in accordance
with the Copyright, Designs and Patents Act 1988.

1 3 5 7 9 8 6 4 2

A CIP catalogue record for this book is available from
the British Library.

Typeset by SetSystems Ltd, Saffron Walden, Essex
Printed and bound in Great Britain by
Mackays of Chatham plc, Chatham, Kent

To my husband
for his
Constancy
Harmony
and
Inspiration

Most people don't get this much love in a lifetime

About the Author

Kathryn Marsden is well known not only as a regular contributor to some of the UK's leading women's magazines but also as the bestselling author of *The Food Combining Diet*, *Food Combining In 30 Days*, *Super Skin* and *The All Day Energy Diet*. She began her research into food combining back in the early 1980s when her husband Ralph was diagnosed with cancer and given only a few weeks to live. Kathryn introduced the diet, together with a range of vitamin and mineral supplements and other alternative therapies, in an effort to make him more comfortable. The six-week deadline came and went. '*After that*,' says Kathryn, '*we greeted every new day as a bonus*.'

Although they never considered food combining as a cure, they both felt that it encouraged some kind of inner healing. It was especially helpful following the extensive surgery to remove Ralph's stomach and spleen. His digestion and energy levels, at an all-time low after the two massive operations, only improved when food combining and a programme of vitamin and mineral supplements were introduced. The cancer went into remission and a few weeks became months and then years.

In fact, Ralph lived *twelve more years*, but when he fell ill again in 1995 decided that he didn't want to go on. '*He asked me to promise him that I wouldn't be miserable. I said*

*I couldn't promise but I would do my best. Of course, there were
bad days and good days. We'd been such good pals and I missed
his crazy Liverpool humour. I threw myself into work, completed
another manuscript, decorated the house and, as indoor and
outdoor plants are a major hobby, went completely bananas at
the local garden centre! It turned out to be great therapy! People
have been so kind. The support I've had from friends, colleagues,
former patients and readers has touched me deeply and given me
the incentive to keep my chin up.'*

On a personal level, Kathryn assumed, quite contentedly,
that she would spend the rest of her life unattached. *'No one
could have been more surprised than I was when I fell head over
heels for a friend of Ralph's whom I'd already known for more
than twenty years. No, not a rebound, but a contented and comfortable friendship with lots of deep affection. Richard had been
on his own for nearly a decade but we'd never taken the slightest
interest in each other. We went out together a few times just for company. Then something clicked and we realized we were thoroughly
miserable when we were apart. We took a holiday in America in
October 1996 and, while we were away, he proposed. Take it from
me that romance is alive and well in the over-40s! Apart from the
fact that we are both ecstatically happy, the great thing is that we
know Ralph would be really pleased we're together.*

*'We both enjoy following a food-combining diet, usually for
five days a week, and have complete faith in its principles. I've
seen so many people benefit and, even now, get stacks of letters
from readers who tell me how well it works for them.'*

Kathryn and Richard were married in April 1997. They
share a cottage in deepest Wiltshire with various rescued
cats and a variety of other welcome wildlife.

The Food Combining 2-Day Detox

Contents

ॐ

Foreword

❦

Did you know that last year alone in the UK, we drank 200 million alcoholic drinks, smoked 83 billion cigarettes, downed one million tons of food chemicals and swallowed 50,000 tons of antibiotics? Over 450 million prescriptions were written for a variety of medicines. Four hundred million litres of pesticides were sprayed over our fruits, vegetables and grains. And untold quantities of polluted air were added to our toxic overload.

It has been estimated that only around 3% of the world's population actually eat a healthy balanced diet; the rest of us may talk about health, but carry on eating junk. Could one of the main reasons for the tidal wave of degenerative illness we have today be that our bodies have had enough?

During my teens, I suffered dreadfully from chronic throat infections, acne and glandular fever, for which I was prescribed a variety of medicines, including almost continuous antibiotics. As teens passed into twenties, the legacy of so many drugs triggered candida and, eventually, chronic fatigue. My immune system and digestion were wrecked by year upon year of stress and poor diet. I struggled on, always tired, never fit – but it never occurred to me that I could help myself – until

I met Kathryn Marsden. That was almost twenty years ago.

Kathryn guided me towards a totally new, far healthier way of eating that, slowly but surely, helped me back to health. One of the most important things I learned is the need to regularly clean up the system and reduce the body's constantly accumulating toxic burden. None of it was difficult and I have benefited beyond measure. Never did I dream that, one day, I would have my own health column in a national newspaper. But now I have, and in no small part thanks to Kathryn Marsden.

I know that Kathryn's fundamental aim in all her work is that food should be *enjoyable* as well as good for us. *The Food Combining 2-Day Detox* has nothing whatever to do with difficult diets or deprivation. I hope that you will find, as I did, that her sound advice encourages you to look more closely at your food choices and to take more care of yourself. If you do, I think you'll feel more energized than you have for years.

Kathryn is a leading light in modern nutritional therapy. After a decade in clinical practice, she now writes regularly for a whole range of magazines and journals, and has several best-selling books to her name. Read *The Food Combining 2-Day Detox* and you'll see why!

Hazel Courteney
'What's the Alternative?'
The Sunday Times

Introduction

⋊⋋

> Married women are taught that if they wish to get
> along with their mate they should 'feed the brute' on
> the assumption that only when the stomach is full is
> a man in good temper!
>
> *Dr William Howard Hay, 1934*

The Food Combining 2-Day Detox is a book about feeling
  better. *Heaps better*.
It's about feeding your body more healthily.
It's a book for women, written by a woman who *truly*
  understands how you feel.
And it's for anyone who is fed up with feeling lousy,
  lethargic or just low.

If podgy, bloated or bog-eyed fits the bill—
If you're stressed beyond belief—
If you sigh a lot—
If your skin is suffering and
  You're fed up with orange-peel thighs—
If you or your bowel are irritable—
If you're fed up with fighting the flab—
If you feel ratty, fancy a good whinge or are just harassed
  out of your head and hacked off with life in general—

Then *The Food Combining 2-Day Detox* is designed to lift you out of the doldrums – effortlessly and without complication.

Not only is a regular dietary 'clean-up' good preventative medicine, it can be especially important if your health has been under any kind of strain.

For example?

Detoxification is one of the best ways of chasing a cold away. Page 14 has details. It's also a great way to wake up a tired body, lift the lethargy caused by too many late nights or compensate for a period of over-indulgence! If you need to lose a little weight but nothing you've done so far has made any long-term difference, *The Food Combining 2-Day Detox* could be just the thing to shake up a sluggish metabolism.

These two-day sessions aren't difficult to do and, if repeated regularly, are far more beneficial to the body than paying homage to all that awful post-Christmas and pre-holiday deprivation-dieting that so many people seem to slog through.

Apart from anything else, you'll be better nourished. Compared to the average 1000-calorie low-fat diet, this food-combining programme offers far better balance, providing nutrient-dense sustenance, the right level of daily dietary fibre and plenty of rehydrating fluid. You won't be bothered by hunger pangs either. There is far too much delicious food here for that to happen!

But why the need for DETOX at all? The human body already has a number of sophisticated mechanisms for ridding itself of unwanted wastes. Surely the system is automatic?

Unfortunately, the time-saving trappings of the modern twentieth-century lifestyle mean that we are taking in more pollutants and producing more metabolic debris than our 'in-house' garbage-disposal systems can cope with.

Very few of us eat an ideal diet. We consume mass-produced, processed and denatured convenience food, artificial colours, flavours and preservatives (many made from coal tar or petrochemical derivatives). There are over-the-counter and prescription medicines; drug, pesticide and hormone residues in our food and water supply, and industrial emissions and traffic exhaust fumes to deal with, too. DDT (banned but still around and causing concern), dioxins and heavy metals are seen as particularly serious problems.

Just as a matter of interest, it's been estimated that the air in most large towns and cities is so polluted that even non-smokers are sucking in the equivalent of 40 cigarettes per day.

Collectively all these factors put pressure on a body that one could hardly claim was designed to cope, since it hasn't evolved much in the last ten thousand years. Add all this to lack of exercise, inadequate rest and negative stress, and there seems little doubt but that the system is struggling.

When elimination processes slow down, skin becomes rough and sallow, and hair is lifeless. The liver and kidneys – two main routes of rubbish recycling – are on overtime. Bowels get sluggish. We breathe less deeply and pump less oxygen so that fewer nutrients are delivered to where they are needed, and poisons hang around for too long in the bloodstream. The nutrients that *are* available are used up far too quickly, leaving the body less resistant to infection and more prone to free radical damage. (See page 74 for more about free radicals.)

Is it any wonder that energy slumps and we don't feel so great?

Of course, you and I would be the first to agree that the over-zealous toxin seeker can find potentially undesirable chemicals in almost everything. Household cleaning fluids, carpets, cosmetics, toothpaste, tap water, paint and plastic packaging, to name but a few. It could be extremely easy to get paranoid about the poisons that invade our everyday lives.

But they are there. And most of them have been in use only for a very short time – in the case of some new chemicals, perhaps a generation or less. So we don't yet know what long-term effects they have on us. And it's nigh impossible to avoid them.

There is, however, ample clinical evidence to demonstrate that short periods (in this case, a day or two at most) on super-fresh, energy-packed, vitamin-rich produce can give a tired, stressed, overworked, undernourished body a cleansing, immune-boosting, health-enhancing, mood-lifting tonic.

Cleansing diets come in all shapes and sizes. Some are very restrictive, allowing only vegetable and fruit juices. Others follow the mono-diet therapy of using just one kind of fruit and nothing else for several days: for example, grapes, apples or grapefruit. In certain circumstances, properly supervised, these recommendations can be extremely beneficial. However, they require a full understanding of what is involved, proper supervision, dedication, a lot of resolve and, of course, time. Previous health history and any current medication must be taken into account because restricting food intake is contraindicated in certain conditions, for example, diabetes or pregnancy.

> He that eats till he is sick must fast till he is well.
>
> *Old Hebrew proverb*

Fasting and the avoidance of solid food have a strong association with both medical and religious practices, as a way of cleansing the body and focusing the mind.

Clinics that specialize in the treatment of alcohol or drug dependence will often recommend using a diet-based detoxification treatment as part of the recovery programme. Such procedures can be helpful in any kind of addiction but don't necessarily need to be rigorous or rigid in order to work. For example, some of the simple basics outlined in this book have helped people quit smoking, deal with comfort eating and kick the sugar-craving habit.

The problem is that when you're exhausted, depressed or plagued by hypoglycaemia (low blood sugar) – and you haven't had time to eat, doughnuts and chocolate seem somehow so much more attractive than internal cleansing. Very few people under any circumstances would wax enthusiastic about lemon juice, lettuce leaves or cabbage water.

But if you think that's what this book is about, you'd be wrong.

The *Food Combining 2-Day Detox* is an entirely different approach and is designed especially:

For women who, like me, work long hours and have little, if any, free time

For people who feel that their lives are under siege and

For those who have no immediately serious health problems but are plagued by, perhaps, premenstrual cramps, bloating, skin eruptions, flaking nails, constipation, dark circles around the eyes, a furry tongue, aches and

pains or just vague, niggly symptoms that are difficult
to describe.

If you're interested in
  Putting a spring in your step
  Lifting your spirits and
  Eating more healthily in the long-term
If you'd like to say a fond farewell to cellulite
If you hanker after younger-looking skin
  Stronger nails and glossier hair
  Improved circulation
  Better digestion and elimination
  Better weight control and
  More energy

Then introduce the Food Combining 2-Day Detox *into your
life.*

No, it's not a quick fix, or a miracle cure, but a healthy
way to encourage better body function.

WOMEN are particularly at risk from stress, overwork and
undernourishment. Along with emancipation, alleged
equality and a certain amount of independence, women
have also maintained the right to be terminally exhausted.
If you have children, a home to keep going, school runs to
do, a husband or partner to feed, parents or elderly
relatives to look out for, or anything else that eats into
your space, you'll know exactly how that feels. If you have
a full-time job and no leisure in your own life, who is

going to care whether you ate pot noodles and fries on the run or burped your way through brown rice and beans, how well you slept or how much carbon monoxide you breathed in on the road to the supermarket?

Well, I do – and your body certainly will.

The time has come to nurture yourself a little.

This book is not about deprivation. There's no pressure or guilt here. Nor is it necessary to introduce the *unusual* or the *weird* or the *impossible to follow* in order to succeed. An occasional internal clean-up and body-pampering session offers enormous health benefits.

The *Food Combining 2-Day Detox* is for anyone who *really, seriously*, would love to feel fitter but doesn't have the inclination – or the hours in a day – to fit anything else whatsoever into their lives.

You, too?

The enemy is always *Time*, isn't it? So, to a certain extent, I guess, is commitment. Maybe we choose to vegetate rather than meditate because we see looking after ourselves, our personal selves, as some kind of treat we don't have time for – or don't deserve. We assume our own needs are right at the bottom of that long, long list of other priorities. At the end of the day, we have no steam left to take any interest in anything new. The cop-out is simpler. Simply don't bother. Who needs bowel-washing, beds of nails and all that humming, anyway?

There are already plenty of books out there telling us how easy it is to lose weight, eat the right food, clean our colons, improve our health, love our bodies and expand our minds. The problem is that most of us don't have a spare minute even to read about it, let alone to put any of it into practice. And yet, with only the smallest effort, it is possible to reconnect with that almost forgotten feeling of wellbeing.

So what's here that's different?

Well, first up you'll find out why detoxification is so important to our long-term health (no boring technical details, I promise); then I'll tell you how making a few changes to your existing diet can work wonders for the way your body behaves.

No extremes or hard regimes, just commonsense health advice and some humour to go along with it.

You probably feel tired at the moment – maybe too tired to be bothered – but hang in here and prepare to be amazed. I've done all of this for myself, too, and believe me, it makes such a difference!

To encourage and maintain the improvements, I'll be giving you the easiest of all introductions to food combining. If you've been there, seen or had a go at any kind of food combining before, you might have given up because you thought it was complicated, you didn't understand it, or perhaps you just drifted back into old habits.

It's easily done. No need to lose any Brownie points for that. We've all fallen into the same trap.

But Kathryn Marsden's kind of food combining is so easy to follow. It has proved itself to be one of the most enjoyable and painless ways to improve body function and, where necessary, to encourage healthy weight loss.

Since *The Food Combining Diet* topped the bestseller lists, other books have jumped on the bandwagon. But without clinical experience or genuine understanding of food-combining basics, some explanations are unnecessarily complicated, confusing and unfortunately not always accurate.

If you've never tried my kind of food combining before, you could be very pleasantly surprised. As a practitioner, I've received an enormous amount of feedback from patients on how this hassle-free system has helped improve their health, often in situations where nothing else had worked. Other practitioners receive similar reports. My book *Food Combining In 30 Days* contains extracts from just a few of the letters I've received. (I forgive and feel sorry for the misguided researcher of a particular television programme who tried to suggest that I made them up! What would be the point?)

The correspondence keeps on coming! From all over the world! A typical example is a recent letter from Spain. A delightful lady, 35 years old, writes to me to say that she had suffered for years feeling uncomfortable, bloated and sluggish, with hormone problems and troublesome skin. *'Three months into food combining and my body is functioning like it has never done before. All those years of lost energy have come back and my skin is getting better by the day. And "hooray", I can wear nearly my whole wardrobe again. I feel re-born.'*

I hope you enjoy reading *The Food Combining 2-Day Detox*. I hope, even more, that you have some fun putting its principles into practice and reaping its benefits. Do as much or as little as you feel you have time for but, above all, *enjoy the experience.*

And if, at any stage, your life is going through a bad patch and things are a bit rough, delight in the sentiment which prompted this observation:

When God made man, she was having one of her off days.

Never forget how important it is to nurture *yourself* sometimes.

Wishing you love, light, laughter and better health.

Kathryn Marsden
Wiltshire, England

Is Detox a Dirty Word?

ༀ

At no point in the course of study does the medical
student receive any sound and organised instruction
in the field of nutrition: he has to depend on (little
more than) scrappy gossip.

Sir Walter Fletcher
Secretary of the Medical Research Council of Great Britain
at Pennsylvania University, 1930

AUTHOR'S NOTE: In conversations with three GPs, I have been
advised that the amount of nutritional study currently provided
to medical students during their seven-year training period
varies from 'sixty minutes' or 'about half a day' to 'twelve hours
or so'.

It's an unfortunate thing about the word 'detox' that it
nearly always conjures pictures of pain and self-denial,
going without food for days on end, drowning in the
discipline of drinking a dozen litres of water, bathing in
Epsom salts, taking endless enemas or, worse still, suffering the colonic-irrigating indignity of having freezing-
cold metal nozzles and long plastic tubes of the kind
that are fixed to the outlets of externally vented tumble
dryers shoved up one's backside. Joking apart, properly

supervised by a qualified practitioner, colonic irrigation –
and fasting – can have enormous health benefits.

A true fast means eating no solid foods and surviving for
a period of several days or weeks on water alone. Taking
only juices or fruit is a stringent method of detoxification
and is, in truth, a juice or fruit 'cure'. It is not a fast.
Scientific research shows that both methods can be beneficial to a range of diseases that includes pancreatitis,
schizophrenia, arthritis, cardiovascular problems, inflammation and infection of the kidneys, and eczema and other
skin disorders. Unfortunately, though, the very word
'fasting' has come to represent one of the more fanatical
and inflexible facets of dieting. You know the kind of
thing. Yogis do it on a budget to reach a higher
consciousness; the weight-conscious wealthy do it in style
and pay heaps of money for the privilege.

But don't confuse fasting with simple detoxification
programmes of short duration that actually encourage an
increased intake of particular types of food and fluid.

Case-history studies suggest that the type of detox programme I am showing you here works in several ways.
First of all, the strain is taken off the digestive system,
encouraging it to work more efficiently. Patients who
suffered digestive and bowel disorders say they have better
elimination and less discomfort. In many cases, symptoms
disappeared completely.

Secondly, because digestion is easier, foods are dealt
with more effectively and more nutrients are absorbed.

Those who complained of constant colds and recurring infections demonstrated far better resistance after using food combining in conjunction with two-day cleansing. Other listed benefits include improved sleep pattern and more energy throughout the day, stronger nails and improved skin condition. There is no doubt in my mind that detoxification and simple dietary improvements are key elements in recovery.

For minor complaints such as a cold or hangover, a day on juices and water kicks the immunity into gear and gives the digestive system a holiday. See page 14.

Despite these encouragements, there will always be those who disagree that detoxification is therapeutic.

For or Against?

Detractors deride DETOX as
  Dangerous mythology
  Encouraging Eating disorders
  Treacherous and Troublesome
  Obsessive and
  eXtreme.

Experts who sneer at the need for detoxification say that the whole notion is nonsense. Detoxing, they contend, *could be harmful to the body.*

But aren't toxins themselves harmful?

Take just one toxic problem: pesticide residues. Apparently, these particular poisons are stored '*relatively harmlessly*' (excuse me?) in human fat tissue. Trying to get rid of them *too quickly* '*might*' be damaging.

> TOXIN is a general term used to describe any kind of poison. Accurately, 'toxins' include poisons produced by micro-organisms within the body, such as the extremely dangerous E. coli bacteria responsible for the Scottish food-poisoning outbreaks. Also covered are farm chemicals, industrial wastes and the gases produced by cigarettes and vehicle exhausts. 'Toxin' has fallen into common usage, describing the accumulation of chemicals and other pollutants that enter the body via the food and water supply or from the air that we breathe. 'Detoxification', or 'detox', is the term used to describe a natural method of inner cleansing.

First of all we are persuaded that detoxification is unnecessary because the body gets rid of unwanted wastes and chemicals *without our help*. But then official sources acknowledge that organophosphates (pesticides known to cause a whole range of horrendous symptoms as well as being implicated in brain degeneration and immune system disorders) are alive and well in our fat cells.

But it's OK, apparently, because they are 'relatively' harmless.

That would be . . . um . . . relative to what, exactly?

The evidence is already there to show that pesticide residues and other pollutants are causing havoc with our health and our environment. Various authorities (agrochemical manufacturers among them) assure us that there is nothing to worry about, but they cannot know how the human body will cope with these alien intrusions in the long term. As Graham Harvey points out in his book *The Killing of the Countryside*, science knows virtually nothing about the dangers of prolonged exposure. Fears about the potentially damaging effects of farm chemicals are far from irrational and are underpinned by a growing weight of evidence.

LET'S TAKE A BRIEF LOOK AT HOW ACCURATE AGRI-CULTURAL INDUSTRY AND GOVERNMENT PLATITUDES MIGHT BE.

An accusing finger has been pointing in the direction of organophosphates for several years and yet it is only now, following several damning reports (including one suggesting a likely link to BSE), that officialdom is beginning to take notice.

Various tests show pesticide residues at unacceptable levels in a range of foods; between 20 per cent and

33 per cent of fruits and vegetables in sampling contained contaminants in excess of the government's MRLs (Maximum Residue Levels).

When staples such as bread, potatoes and milk were tested, one third to one half of the examples were considered well above safe limits.

In one case, a lettuce was found to be 45 *times* the maximum 'safe' limit for a fungicide known as dithiocarbamate.

Most commercially grown lettuces are estimated to be sprayed around 25 times during their life cycle with one or more agrochemicals.

Chocolate samples revealed 82 per cent were tainted with the pesticide Lindane (banned in several countries but, at the time of writing, still permitted in the UK).

And, by the way, these percentages don't mean that the rest of foods tested were pesticide-free – just that they were within the maximum limits allowed!

Rotten to the Core?

The ability of some pesticides to penetrate the whole vegetable or fruit was highlighted by a Ministry of Agriculture report which agreed that testing just the peel or skin alone *was likely to seriously underestimate the actual amounts of chemicals being consumed by the public*. In other words, peeling the produce won't necessarily protect us from contamination. Indeed, it seems that because of the systemic nature of these chemicals, we are probably swallowing far higher doses than had previously been supposed.

PESTICIDES COULD BE RESPONSIBLE FOR BRITTLE BONES.

The most recent news is that one kind of OP (organophosphate) may be responsible for another OP – osteoporosis. New evidence suggests that, apart from all their other misdemeanours, organophosphates might be at least one trigger for the worrying increase in fragile bones. Further investigations are urgently needed. The National Osteoporosis Society is quoted as saying that 'the insignificant funding for this type of research is a scandal.' (See page 18 for more on pesticides.)

Several other organizations, the prestigious Royal Society for the Protection of Birds among them, have also expressed serious disquiet about the indirect but permanent damage that is caused by farm and industrial chemicals in the food chain. As with the investigation into Gulf War Syndrome (for several years denied a proper hearing on the basis that thousands of servicemen were all imagining their symptoms), there is concern that researchers have so far bothered themselves only with the quantities of chemicals that might kill or cause immediate and severe disability. No one has taken much interest in the possibility that regular or even one-off ingestion of small amounts of toxins might create serious illness over the long term.

A Pinch of Salt

Comforting edicts about last year's toxins already being long gone from the system without needing any help from detoxification treatments should be considered carefully.

A good example?

ANTIBIOTICS CAN CAUSE SKIN PROBLEMS FOR MANY MONTHS AFTER THE COURSE HAS BEEN COMPLETED.

It is well known that antibiotics and sun exposure don't always mix, causing skin eruptions, sores, boils and blisters in sensitive individuals. But did you know that someone can still be affected by skin problems in the sun even if their last prescription for antibiotics was up to two years prior to that exposure? That's because the residues of the drug remain in the tissues for a very long time.

NOW THERE MAY BE A PESTICIDE LINK BETWEEN OPs AND CFS?

Still more research has discovered a connection between the delayed onset of Chronic Fatigue Syndrome and previous exposure to pesticides. It is only very recently that the medical profession has acknowledged that Myalgic Encephalomyelitis (also known as Chronic Fatigue Syndrome) is a genuine physical illness. Some doctors still deny it exists. Others say it is all in the mind. I have seen many patients suffering, very genuinely, from this condition. It is interesting that so many have found food-combining programmes helpful during their recovery.

Avoiding Excesses and Extremes

A major objection levelled at detoxification is that it leads to anorexia. A justifiable concern? It is most certainly the case that trying to clean up the system by following any kind of extreme crash diet could not only put enormous strain on the liver and the kidneys but might indeed encourage eating disorders. Of course, fasting should never be recommended to potential anorexics and especially not to teenagers trying to emulate emaciated models. Unfortunately, the human animal, for all its alleged sophistication, has a very unhealthy habit of taking all manner of things to ridiculous extremes.

I have to say that I think responsibility for creating an environment in which eating disorders flourish lies far more fairly and squarely at the doors of the diet-food industry and those sections of the media who persist in portraying skin-and-bone body images instead of real people. You might have noticed that the model on the front cover of *this* book and the model on the front cover of *The All Day Energy Diet* are both shapely and padded, not skinny or undernourished.

But let's not confuse uncontrolled or irresponsible fasting with the tried and tested dietary methods recommended here. Used in conjunction with healthier eating habits – and, where necessary, with herbal remedies and vitamin and mineral supplements – the *Food Combining*

2-Day Detox could be an important step in providing the body with at least some protection against the constant onslaught of what have become known as 'twentieth-century toxins'.

Important, too, is the need to reduce as much as possible our exposure to toxic pollutants. The chapter entitled 'Long-term Protection' which begins on page 16 has advice on how to reduce the overload.

For, Not Against

Enthusiasts see DETOX as
   Definitely **D**esirable
   Efficacious, **E**ffective, **E**asy-to-follow
   Time-honoured, **T**ried, **T**ested and producing
   Outstanding and
   e**X**ceptional results!

Some of the most celebrated names in medicine, science, nutrition and naturopathy have researched and written about the benefits to the body of controlled fasting and inner cleansing.

Many of them can relate some remarkable case histories! Dr Max Bircher-Benner, Dr Norman Walker, Dr Herbert Shelton, Max Gerson and the eminent Swiss doctor H.C.A. Vogel could be considered the early twentieth-century gurus of natural health care, followed by the renowned

practitioners and health writers of today such as Dr
Bernard Jensen, Annemarie Colbin, Leslie Kenton, Jan de
Vries, Celia Wright, Leon Chaitow, Dr John Briffa,
Gillian Hamer and Harald Gaier, adviser and columnist
to the groundbreaking journals *What Doctors Don't Tell
You* and *Proof!*

While some authorities are emphatic that detoxification
is entirely unnecessary, there will be other practitioners
and health experts who say that the type of programme
recommended here is not stringent enough. That may be
so for some people. However, detoxing using water and
lemon juice only could prove too drastic and debilitating
for those who need to eat regularly to maintain energy
levels. In my experience with patients, that could be
the majority of us. Going without food, even for short
periods of time, can cause massive swings in blood-glucose
levels, encouraging hypoglycaemic symptoms such as
poor coordination, lack of concentration, a fall in body
temperature, hot or cold sweats, stomach pains and
dizziness.

In addition, the way in which toxic debris from our
modern environment accumulates in our fat cells means
that we should take particular care over how it is removed.

Let me explain.

During detoxification, fat is broken down and mobilized
into the bloodstream. Along with it go a whole heap of
stored chemicals. In a very toxic body (again, that's
probably most of us), long-term cleansing can cause too

many toxins to be released at once, leading to unpleasant reactions, similar to those that might occur if a range of rather nasty poisons were injected directly into the bloodstream from a syringe!

This is just one more reason why a gentle system of short-term but regular detoxification has many benefits over longer and less flexible 'regimes', helping slowly to reduce the overload and protecting against future build-up. In addition, periodic two- or three-day detoxification is an excellent way to:

- Improve digestion and absorption of vital nourishment.
- Stir a sluggish bowel into life and get rid of solid wastes.
- Keep blood glucose in balance.
- Lift lethargy and give a feeling of general wellbeing.
- Encourage healthier eating habits.
- Improve the health of the skin, hair and nails.
- There have also been several reports of better breathing, lessened allergic reactions and fewer colds.

The *Food Combining 2-Day Detox* is based on sound naturopathic principles but I make no apologies for presenting it in a less stringent though none-the-less effective format.

Introduce the programme any time you have time. Once or twice a month is about right. Less often is also good — and better than not doing it at all. It doesn't matter whether you choose week days or weekends, but try to organize your personal routine so that you have a little less stress around you and not so much pressure from other people.

Want to do More?

For those who prefer a slightly more strict detox programme, a third day is recommended (see page 111). However, don't introduce Day Three unless you are able to take time off and rest properly.

On page 14, you'll find a JUICE-ONLY DETOX DAY designed specifically for anyone who is suffering from a cold or has *really* pushed alcohol or rich food to excess! Taking nothing more than fruit and vegetable juices or plain vegetable broth for one day gives the digestive system a complete rest, allowing detoxification to take place without hindrance and pushing the body's energy into boosting the immune system.

These kinds of fluids on their own contain relatively little in the way of dietary fibre. Something not to be recommended, you might think. However, the digestive system has to work much harder when it is dealing with roughage, especially the insoluble cereals. Juices, on the other hand, provide easily absorbed vitamins and minerals without the need for extensive digestion.

The food-combining guidelines which begin on page 47 and the tips and hints on pages 53 to 61 are there to help you too. Introduce them one at a time into your *everyday* eating habits to enhance the overall quality and nourishment value of the food you choose; a kind of long-term 'health insurance' which hopefully increases resistance to illnesses (such as cardiovascular and digestive disorders) that have a known diet connection.

A stuffed stomach makes for a dull head and a foggy brain.

The JUICE-ONLY ONE-DAY DETOX described here can ease the misery of a cold. It is also extremely soothing and forgiving to anyone who has eaten too much or over-indulged on alcohol the day before. If you do not have a cold and are using the recommendations to calm a stressed digestion, follow the same programme, but substitute Boldocynara tincture for the Echinaforce. For more information on Boldocynara, see the chapter on Looking After Your Liver which begins on page 70.

- At the first sign of symptoms, take a hot bath, using a few drops of essential oil of Ginger in the bath water. Wrap up warm and go to bed. Put three drops of Eucalyptus and three of Lemon Grass in a vaporizer in the bedroom. See page 120 for essential info on essential oils.
- Introduce a mini-detox by taking fresh fluids, such as fruit and vegetable juices or vegetable broth and water,

for 24 hours. For this one day, forget about solid foods. (See the note on page 97 about liquid foods.)

- Take a 1-gram tablet or capsule of a low acid/buffered Vitamin C Complex every three hours. Also take 30 drops of echinacea tincture (Echinaforce is available from health stores) in a little water three times a day. You should find that this reduces symptoms and cuts down the duration of the cold. In some cases, if done quickly enough, it can knock the virus on the head immediately!

No one really knows why this method works but experts guess that, because the digestion has less work to do, the body is able to put all its effort into supporting the immune system. Once you are out of bed, stay on a light diet for a few days and continue taking 2 grams of Vitamin C every day and the Echinaforce (or Boldocynara) until the bottle is empty. If you are plagued with a sore throat, catarrh or sinusitis, add a daily capsule or tablet of garlic to your supplements. See page 139 for info on how to find local stockists for these products.

Long-term Protection – Reducing Exposure to Toxins

჻

჻

Woman is not needed to do man's work. She is not needed to think man's thoughts (nor) to enhance masculine spirit but to express the feminine. Hers is not to preserve a man-made world but to create a human world by the infusion of the feminine element into all of its activities.

Margaret Sanger, Woman and The New Race

Just as important as a regular internal spring-clean is the need to reduce exposure to the pollutants and chemicals that contribute to toxicity in the first place. This means being a little more vigilant about the food we eat and the household products we buy. But before you make any changes, consider the thought-provoking facts in the box below.

Worth thinking about?

Organic foods have been found to have two to three times the vitamin and mineral value of chemically raised 'equivalents'.

Organically managed farmland supports more wildlife (including birds) than chemically managed land.

Organic farmers have better sperm counts.

Farmers who use organophosphates suffer from more psychiatric and nervous-system disorders and greater loss of mental skills than those who are not exposed.

Organophosphates are neurotoxic chemicals originally developed as nerve gases.

Studies are now being urged into a possible association between organophosphate contamination and osteoporosis {brittle-bone disease}. The National Osteoporosis Society is concerned that the marked increase in fractures may be being caused by pesticide poisoning.

Researchers who discovered a connection between organ-ophosphates and Chronic Fatigue Syndrome (ME) have also found that there is a long delay between the exposure to the pesticide and the onset of the illness.

Biologists have linked the presence of a number of pesti-cides and hormone residues in the environment to feminization and infertility of male birds, alligators, fish and turtles. Studies show that even the minutest ex-posure to these chemicals, far less than is known to cause cancer, is sufficient to damage reproduction in animals. Researchers are concerned that humans may be similarly affected.

The annual US production of synthetic pesticides exceeds 600,000 tons. This figure *does not include* herbicides, fungicides, fertilizers and other crop chemicals.

Out of 426 commonly used chemicals listed in one toxolog-ical survey, 68 were found to be carcinogenic, 61 could mutate human genes, 35 were found to adversely affect reproduction and 93 caused skin irritations.

Watersports enthusiasts are at risk of stomach upsets and other more serious symptoms if they come into contact with lake and river water during their outdoor activities.

For the real lowdown on how chemical warfare and other damage wrought to the countryside by modern farming practices is destroying the natural balance of nature, read

The Killing of the Countryside by Graham Harvey. (See Recommended Reading on page 149.)

Remember that you can remove a slug or a greenfly from your cabbage but you can't 'pick off' agrichemicals.

Going Organic

Wherever possible, choose organic produce over commercially grown foods. Some areas operate a 'veggie box' scheme. Run by local growers of organic produce, the service aims to make ecologically acceptable food available at affordable prices. Although not so geared up in isolated and rural areas, doorstep deliveries of locally produced organic fruits and vegetables are increasing in towns and cities. Contact the Soil Association (see page 147), who can advise you of your nearest suppliers.

• If organic options are not available or you feel that supermarket organics are beyond your budget, don't give up on fruits and vegetables.

It's true that pesticide residues cannot be totally removed by washing – or even by peeling. However, the benefits may still outweigh the disadvantages. Some wise mathematician once estimated that it's fifteen times better to eat the commercially grown non-organic produce than it is to avoid fruits and vegetables altogether just because they've been sprayed.

- Whatever your source of supply and whether organic or not, wash all fruits, vegetables and salad foods thoroughly. It's not well publicized but bacteria, just as deadly as those implicated in food poisoning caused by poultry, meats and soft cheeses, are also found on other produce including melons, tomatoes, mushrooms and lettuces. Even if you intend to remove the peel or outer leaves on any vegetable or fruit, *wash it thoroughly first.*
- Don't buy foods from roadside stalls. They are not always locally grown or organic. Even if they are not contaminated with pesticide, herbicide or fungicide residues, they could be laced with the fallout from vehicle exhaust emissions.

Dioxins

As far as possible, avoid cow's milk and meat products unless they are organic. Apart from the inevitable concerns about BSE, these foods are also common sources of dioxin residues.

Dioxins are toxic by-products of the chlorine-bleach and paper-pulp industries and are given off during chemical reprocessing and medical waste incineration. They then 'fall out' from the atmosphere and settle on grass land which is eaten by farm animals and wildlife. Dioxins are *known* to cause cancer, infertility and birth defects. Apart from household bleach, chlorine is used in the production of disposable nappies, tissues and cleansing pads, loo rolls, sanitary protection and even some teabags. Other toxic chemicals such as DDT and Lindane, found in milk, are believed by some practitioners to contribute to a wide range of health problems but are said by government sources to be at 'safe levels'.

As dioxins are most concentrated in animal fats, humans are more likely to consume them by eating meat or dairy products from animals fed on foods that are themselves contaminated. Cow's milk, in particular, is an accurate guide to environmental pollution, both past and present levels, because animals grazing in polluted areas pick up pollutants and pass them down the food chain via their milk.

Dioxins have also been implicated in TSS (toxic shock syndrome), an extremely serious and potentially fatal infection caused by a toxin known as TSST-1, produced in the warm environment of the vagina by the normally harmless bacteria *Staphylococcus aureus*. Women using barrier contraceptives are at increased risk from TSS but the greatest danger of all comes from the use of tampons, which allow bacteria to creep into the bloodstream by drying and ulcerating the vaginal wall. Dioxins have also been implicated as a major cause of endometriosis.

The answer to Dioxins

1 Avoid tampons totally and use the older type of bleach-free cotton sanitary pads.
2 If you feel that you can't manage without tampons,

then make sure that you change them even more frequently than you do at present. And always buy bleach-free products. See page 139 for stockist information. According to Victoria Wood, any very old tampon can be used as an anti-mugging device: stuff it up the nose of a potential attacker and he'll immediately see the error of his ways.

3 Use non-chlorine cleaning products in the home.

4 Cut right back on milk intake or give it up altogether. Or drink only small quantities of organic milk (now available in all major supermarkets).

5 Limit your intake of tea, especially if it is made with bleached teabags.

6 Avoid meat unless it is truly organic. Get your proteins from organic poultry, free-range eggs from birds fed organically, sheep's and goat's milk yoghurt and cheeses, fresh oily fish, organic soya milk and other organic soya products.

7 If you're concerned about the cost of 'going organic', don't be. It's true that produce can be a little more expensive but that depends where you shop. With careful planning, food bills don't need to be higher. We all tend to eat too much protein: there really is no need to eat expensive meat products every day. If you're a vegetarian, you'll know that already. By preparing vegetarian dishes using cheaper ingredients such as beans, brown rice, couscous and fresh organic vegetables, on three or four days of the week, you'll still be well nourished as well as staying within your budget.

Reminder: See page 139 for how to locate organic produce.

Filtered Water

Reduce chemical exposure further by filtering all your tap water. I have used an inexpensive jug filter for several years and find it just as effective as the more complicated plumbed-in systems. Most filters will take out a significant proportion of aluminium, nitrates and chlorine, improving the taste and the quality of tap water.

> *Do remember to change the cartridge regularly; at the very least once a month. Wash the jug out thoroughly between each change.*
> *Don't use water that has been standing for long periods or stored for more than a day either in or out of the fridge. Old cartridges and stale water breed bacteria.*

If you are away from home during the day, either take freshly filtered water with you or buy reputable bottled water. On holiday, I used a small portable water-filter unit. See page 143 for more information on the health benefits of water (my thanks to Kenwood for their help with research into the benefits of water filtration).

Aluminium

As far as possible, keep aluminium out of your life. Not only can it disturb digestion, it's yet another toxin that the body has to deal with. It has also been reported that the relatively small amounts of aluminium to which we are exposed every day are enough to upset the liver and mimic symptoms similar to those associated with alcohol-induced cirrhosis. You'll find aluminium lurking in dried foods such as baking powder, milks and dried soups (as an anti-caking agent), in regular brand toothpastes, dental amalgam, antacid medications, some deodorants and in tap water in some areas of the country. If your cooking pots and pans are light in weight, the chances are they could be aluminium. Stainless steel or glass are healthier options.

Toothpaste

Use a chemical-free herbal/mineral toothpaste. Health-food stores stock a good range. Apart from the aforementioned aluminium, many ordinary toothpastes contain a whole array of chemicals which, although not directly or immediately harmful, may contribute to the build-up of toxicity. There is also some evidence that the foaming agents and detergents (such as sodium laurel sulphate) used in a number of ordinary toothpastes are not removed by mouth rinsing because they actually bind to gum tissue. Formaldehyde, bromchlorophen and chlorhexidin are designed to kill bacteria but they also destroy friendly and helpful flora, upsetting the natural balance. It has been suggested that more dangerous bacteria may remain untouched and unharmed. In addition, there is increasing concern about the long-term effects of fluoride toothpaste and fluoridated water on our health and that of our children. And if that were not enough, it's worth pointing out that the membranes of the mouth are a shortcut route to the bloodstream. That's great for vital substances (sublingual drugs for angina are administered this way; so, too, are some vitamin preparations) but not when it comes to potentially harmful chemicals.

Deodorant

Change to a non-chemical deodorant such as Pitrok or Crystal Spring, both available from health stores. Made from natural mineral salts and entirely free of artificial chemicals, these new-style deodorants stop body odour by killing the bacteria that cause the smell. They are suitable for sensitive skins and a better option than aerosol sprays for anyone who suffers from allergies. After washing, wet the crystal and wipe it under the arms, over soles of feet, in the groin and between the breasts. One pack usually lasts about a year. I've used these products in the hottest of climates, including arid Arizona, sticky Singapore and scorching Northern Australia, and they really do work!

Green Gardening

If you are a gardener, avoid the use of weedkillers and other chemicals. It isn't difficult. I'm a very keen gardener but even distant contact with most garden chemicals makes me feel nauseous. Ever noticed the odour given off by the packaged weedkillers and pesticide products when they are stacked side by side in the garden centre? Even this apparently mild exposure can cause queasiness, smarting eyes or sneezing in some sensitive people. When I took on my third-of-an-acre plot ten years ago, it was mostly field grass, rubble, dandelions, thistles and horsetails. Now it is a colourful collection of shrubs, conifers and herbaceous plants protected with gravel and home-made compost and bark. I prefer to use organic and natural alternatives to chemicals. Because weeding is always done by hand when weeds are small (before they burst seed everywhere), I reckon to spend no more than an hour a month attending to garden 'work'. If you're convinced that chemicals are absolutely necessary, take the greatest care when applying them. Read the instructions carefully (you'd be surprised how many people don't) and use only the smallest amount required for the job. Store chemicals carefully and safely with caps secured, away from heat, sunlight, food, pets and children.

Be Well-informed

Write to the head office of the supermarkets you shop at most regularly and ask to see local managers too. Tell them you want more pesticide-free food and accurate labelling on those foods that are sprayed to give you freedom of choice when buying. Write to your MP and MEP and say the same thing. Politicians and retailers do respond to public pressure. Support the Food Labelling Agenda (FLAG), the consumer pressure group started by the Guild of Health Writers and the Guild of Food

Writers, which is campaigning hard for the right to know what really is in our food. FLAG is concerned that we should have clear, comprehensive and meaningful labelling – in other words, information that we can all understand – on all food and food products. In particular, we should know about any pesticides and other agri-chemicals used in the rearing or growing of produce, whether or not foods are irradiated or genetically engin-eered, and what exactly are the kinds and quantities of hidden fats, sugars, salts and other additives. The address for FLAG is on page 148.

- Subscribe to the *Food Magazine*, published by the Food Commission, a national, independent, not-for-profit organization that campaigns for safer, healthier food. They receive no government subsidies and are not supported by advertising or by the food industry. Write to the Publications Department, The Food Commission, 3rd Floor, 5/11 Worship Street, London EC2A 2BH.

- Read *The Food We Eat* by award-winning author Joanna Blythman and find out how to buy food that you can trust. She writes an especially good chapter on chemically dependent farming and organic alternatives, and how to avoid pesticide residues.

Careful How You Breathe

When refuelling at the gas station, try to avoid breathing deeply and, particularly, breathing directly over the filler. Apart from exhaust emissions spewed out of incoming and outgoing vehicles, fuel vapours give off volatile compounds that are considered by scientists to be potential carcinogens. Unleaded petrol is, it seems, no safer than leaded in this respect.

> 'Nobody is healthy in London; nobody can be.'
> *Mr Woodhouse in Jane Austen's Emma*

- Wherever possible, avoid cigarette smoke, well known as a class-A carcinogen and supplier of toxic by-products! There are, for those who don't know, 100,000,000,000,000 (that's one hundred million million) free radicals in every puff which is why heavy smokers have been found to have five times as many wrinkles as non-smokers. It is estimated that only a few lungfuls of cigarette smoke or similarly polluted air uses up 25mg of Vitamin C. This vital vitamin is just one of many very important antioxidant nutrients that help protect cells against oxidation (cell degeneration) and free-radical damage and, according to studies, could be a major factor in reducing our risk of cancer and heart disease.

Antioxidants

Take a daily antioxidant supplement. Go for a capsule or tablet that contains more than the basic Vitamins A, C and E. Choose a product that includes those three plus the B group (especially B1, B3, B5 and B6) and minerals manganese, selenium and zinc. The Directory on page 139 has details of where to find the best quality.

Improve Diet Quality

Whether you food combine or prefer to stick with mixed meals, stay healthier by *not* relying on these foods too often. The swap sheet on pages 59–60 has a list of tasty alternatives.

Battery or barn eggs – choose eggs from organically fed free-range poultry.

Battery or barn-raised poultry – choose organically fed free-range poultry.

Beef – unless it's truly organic.

Bread – some types are better than others. See Swap Sheet for more information.

Cheeses – avoid those that are coloured, smoked or processed.

Chocolate – choose organic.

Cow's milk – use only small amounts of organic cow's milk.

Coffee – limit to one or two cups maximum daily.

   If you're a coffee addict, try weaning yourself on to grain-based coffee substitutes such as Bioforce Bambu (from health stores). Page 139 has stockist details.

Crisps made with hydrogenated vegetable oils

Diet drinks

Diet foods

Fizzy drinks such as colas

Hydrogenated vegetable oils – always check product labels.

Ice-cream

Low-fat foods containing large numbers of additives

Margarine spreads – buy non-hydrogenated spreads from the health store.

Oranges and orange juice – can cause migraines, headaches and joint pain in some sensitive individuals.

Peanuts

Pork

Refined white flour

Salt and salty foods

Salty snacks

Sugar

Sugar-coated breakfast cereals

Tea – more than three cups per day can rob the body of iron.

Use loose tea wherever possible, avoiding bleached teabags.

Why not introduce some organic herbal or fruit teas as a refreshing alternative?

Wheat-based breakfasts – see Swap Sheet for other suggestions.

A Fond Farewell to Cellulite

꒰

People call me a feminist whenever I express senti-
ments that differentiate me from a doormat.

Rebecca West {1892–1993}

Cellulite is something which very obviously blights the
lives of a great many women but, in the minds of most
skin specialists, remains a mythological absurdity. Even
more fanciful to dermatologists and cosmetic surgeons is
the idea that toxic tissues are, in whole or in part,
responsible for orange-peel skin – or that any kind of
inner cleansing will make it go away.

Despite the fact that you and I know differently, there
is, we are told, nothing wrong with the blood supply to
areas of the body that attract cellulite. So there! The idea
of tissue sludge and stagnant toxins is, apparently, nonsense. There goes that nonsense word again.

Just a thought – but have you noticed how often
the *ex cathedra* dogma about cellulite (rather like the
old chestnut about premenstrual tension) being 'all
in the mind' issues so often out of the mouths of
men?

Practitioners and beauty therapists who treat cellulite see things rather differently. While it is hardly life-threatening, it can be an unsightly nuisance. If it has a bearing upon our health by affecting our self-esteem and body image, that's a good enough reason to want to get rid of it. Cellulite can grip anyone of any age, well-padded, skinny or perfectly formed.

A good friend of mine is an excellent aromatherapist and teacher of new students. When she needs guinea pigs for her massage classes, she will sometimes ask if I'm free to go along. On one occasion, I was assigned to a young student who, only five minutes into the massage, left my side and walked over to my friend. Some whispering went on, whereupon she then returned and completed an excellent treatment. I asked later what was said. 'She came to me,' said the tutor, 'and whispered "no cellulite!". Apparently, she'd never massaged anyone before who didn't have any!' It's interesting that I used to have real orange-peel thighs until I changed my diet and followed the recommendations outlined here!

The actual word 'cellulite' is a misnomer. The condition was discovered – and incorrectly named – about a hundred years ago when doctors thought it was some kind of cellular inflammation. It is now believed to be connected to hormonal changes (wouldn't you just know it had to be hormones!) that encourage cells to become swollen and waterlogged with fluid. The tiny blood vessels near the skin's surface are compressed so that circulation slows down and wastes are not dispersed. The goose-flesh, not surprisingly, feels cold to touch.

If you are prone to cellulite, getting rid of it is not an overnight job. It takes time. Use these tips in conjunction with the *Food Combining 2-Day Detox* and a food-combining maintenance programme as described below.

HERE IS THE PLAN THAT I RECOMMEND TO CONTROL CELLULITE

1 Drink *more* fluid. This may sound contradictory when we've already said that cellulite is linked to trapped fluid – but upping water intake helps circulation, increases blood volume and assists the kidneys in filtering more toxins. Try to down at least six glasses of filtered or bottled water (not fizzy and definitely not chilled) every day, preferably between or before meals. Begin each day with the lemon and honey drink described on page 101.

2 Go in for regular massage. Visits to a qualified aromatherapist contribute to a cleaner system by encouraging better lymph drainage. Sessions are also relaxing and stress-releasing. Stress disturbs the balance of the whole endocrine (hormonal) system, including female hormones. Stress hormones themselves also affect the circulation by causing a thickening of the blood. Anyone who is permanently harassed

and 'hyper' is likely to have slower flowing, more viscous blood than someone who is not generally overanxious.

3 Before bathing, brush the skin, *gently*, with either a loofah or a special skin brush designed for the purpose. Good health stores usually stock them. If you have sensitive skin, choose a soft bristle. If you don't have a brush or loofah, use a clean, dry hand towel instead. {I use the Fill and Foam Long Handled Body Sponge which can be used wet or dry and may be suitable for people with sensitive skins. Available from chemists.} The skin is the largest organ of the body and an efficient eliminator of waste products. However, if dead skin cells are not removed, pores can become clogged and new cells find it more difficult to work their way to the surface. Some skin complaints are believed to be the result of poor elimination of toxins. Skin brushing sloughs off dead skin cells, helps to improve lymph drainage and, of course, stimulates the circulation. I repeat: *Be gentle*. There is no need to make skin sore. Concern yourself only with the areas that you can reach and don't strain or twist the spine trying to cover the whole of the back. Always brush towards the heart.

4 Exfoliate the legs, shoulders, chest (use a soft face cloth on the breasts themselves), arms, hips and abdomen once a week, and the cellulite areas themselves twice a week. One of the best – and least expensive – ways is to use a handful of sea salt mixed with two tablespoons of olive oil. First, take a warm

bath. Then stand up in the water, rub in the salt
mixture, sit down again and wash it off. Even better
rinse off in a cool shower and then rub yourself
vigorously with a warm dry towel. The towel will
pick up a lot of debris and excess oil and should be
washed thoroughly after each use.

Caution: oil can make the bath and shower slippery so take care
when getting in and out.

5 Daily use of aromatherapy oils and good moisturizers
at home are all-important in the cellulite fight. One
of my favourites is to mix 5 drops each of Geranium,
Juniper and Grapefruit pure essential oils into 30ml
(about two tablespoons) of carrier oil. Apricot-kernel
oil is a carrier oil suited to inflamed, sensitive or older
skins. Sweet-almond oil is a carrier oil that is helpful
if you have dry skin. Massage the mixture into
affected areas after every bath or shower. Once you
have dealt with existing cellulite, regular use of oils
and massage helps to keep it at bay. If you prefer not
to mix your own oils, there are several excellent
blends on the market. Page 130 has details of stockists. Page 123 has more information on the use of
essential oils in the home.

6 As a treat, I also use Jurlique Body Contouring Gel.
A combination of active herbal ingredients and
antioxidants, its blurb says that this treatment assists
with the slimming and toning process by dealing
with the build-up of waste matter in the body. I use

it simply as a moisturizer but am delighted with the smoothness of the skin, especially on my arms, legs, thighs and buttocks. Available in the UK and Australia. For details, telephone 0181 995 3948 or write to The Naturopathic Health and Beauty Company, 37 Rothschild Road, Chiswick, London W4 5HT.

7 Breathe more deeply. Done every day, slow, deep breathing relaxes a tense body, reduces stress, encourages sound sleep and improves oxygen flow around the body – all these things help keep skin smooth and well fed. See page 95.

8 Take regular exercise. Again, activity improves circulation and oxygen flow. It is an unfortunate fact of life that cellulite will be worse if you are inactive or spend all day in a sedentary job. Computer-keyboard work and word processing definitely exacerbate cellulite on the hips, thighs and backside!

9 Avoid restrictive underwear, tight jeans, Lycra leggings and pantihose that have very tight waistbands. They all hamper the circulation.

10 Follow the *Food Combining 2-Day Detox* and the course of cleansing herbs described in the chapter on Looking After Your Liver (begins page 70).

If you have tried and failed to beat cellulite before, don't be disheartened. This simple plan *really is worth doing*.

Weight – How to be Diet-wise

꒳

> To be somebody, a woman does not need to be more
> like a man, but simply more of a woman.
>
> *Sally E. Shaywitz*

Most people who are genuinely overweight would agree
that losing some excess baggage makes good health sense.
Everyone knows that obesity (which means being more
than a stone over your ideal weight) increases the risk of
heart disease, diabetes and other serious health disorders.
But what hope is there for those who fight an ongoing
battle with their weight, trying every new diet that comes
along, perhaps succeeding for a while but then slipping
back into old habits? Or maybe you are one of those who
just can't lose weight no matter how you try.

New research is turning up lots of fresh information
about why people who don't eat to excess are overweight
and why they are finding it so hard to lose those stubborn
pounds.

First of all, how heavy we are is much more likely to be
determined by our genetic make-up, individual biochem-
istry, physiology and metabolism than by how much food
we eat. Another very interesting theory is that some

weight problems can be linked to poor digestion and 'internal cellular pollution'. There is particular concern, for example, that our ongoing consumption of artificial food additives (preservatives, sweeteners, colours etc.) may make it more difficult for us to control our weight because of the effect such chemicals have on our liver – the body's major detoxification plant. Apart from these pollutants and others that we take in from our daily diet and environment, there are the wastes created as a result of the normal processes of metabolism.

Although receiving renewed attention, the idea that clogged and congested tissues affect metabolism is not a modern theory. A book written in 1926 by Dr J.H. Tilden, called *Toxaemia Explained*, suggests that these wastes, if allowed to build up, create a kind of internal pollution. When more toxins are accumulated than are eliminated, metabolic rate is disturbed and calorie burning slows down.

One reason why food combining and detoxification work so well together is perhaps because they do so much to improve the internal functioning of the body, particularly of the liver, digestive system and bowel. Nutrients are absorbed and metabolized more efficiently and wastes properly excreted. Interestingly, Dr Tilden was himself an early advocate of the food-combining system.

Don't be disappointed if you put on a pound or two as you approach middle age. It makes excellent health sense for us females to be a little heavier at 50 that we were at 20. A bit of extra padding is Mother Nature's way of helping to keep our endocrine (hormonal) system healthy, reducing menopausal symptoms and providing additional protection against osteoporosis (brittle-bone disease).

If you have symptoms of lethargy, persistent tiredness, depression, constipation, hair loss, reduced or non-existent sex drive, high cholesterol, high blood pressure or dry skin, ask your GP about the possibility of a full blood profile to include all female hormones and a test for thyroid function. Hypothyroidism, the medical term for an underactive thyroid gland and a common cause of weight problems, often goes undetected in standard tests. If you are concerned, ask for TSH (thyroid-stimulating hormone) to be tested as well. Many doctors still only check the levels of thyroid hormone circulating in the blood, a test that doesn't always pick up signs of a sluggish thyroid. The condition contributes to obesity by slowing the metabolic rate so that fewer and fewer calories are burned off, *irrespective of how much you eat or how much you exercise.*

Don't Diet – Food-combine Instead

Interestingly, food combining was never designed as a weight-loss diet. The original concept was a healthy-eating programme that encouraged inner cleansing and healing, resistance against illness and enhanced wellbeing. The bonus was that it stimulated slow but sound and sensible weight loss – even in people who had not previously been successful in losing weight – without the need to follow crash diets or drastically cut food intake.

Persistent on-off dieting for weight loss can be a very dangerous pastime and is known to increase the risk of a number of disorders, including hormonal imbalances, gallbladder disease and heart problems.

If you are only two or three pounds over your ideal weight, don't diet. Your bodyweight can vary daily by this amount – it's down to when you weigh yourself. Indeed, unless you are more than half a stone overweight, it really is healthier to go up a dress size than to risk your long-term health by putting yourself through endless dieting deprivation.

If you really feel you need to lose weight, one of the best ways is first to follow the *Food Combining 2-Day Detox* and then to introduce the food-combining hints (see pages 52–61) for 30 days or so. If you honestly need to lose more weight after this, then follow food-combining principles for four or five days each week. This pattern should help you to shed around one kilo (2 pounds) a week. Lose the flab more quickly than this and it will almost certainly creep back.

Kathryn Marsden's Hints to Help Healthy Weight Loss

- Make a shopping list and stick to it. The temptation to buy items on impulse is reduced and you won't over-stock the refrigerator or cupboards. Shop *after* meals, not when you're hungry. That way, you're more likely to buy only what you need.
- Instead of choosing packaged foods, check to see if the fresh equivalents are available. The benefits? More nourishment, fewer additives – so fewer toxins – and, probably, less expense!
- Drink plenty of water between meals and another glass ten minutes before each meal. If you're flagging and aren't able to eat, a glass of water can help to stave off hunger pangs.
- If you suffer from 'water weight' or bloating, drinking more can actually help to reduce fluid retention. Try also to cut down on salt. It has a nasty habit of hanging on to water and may aggravate weight prob-lems even if the diet is otherwise perfect. Give food more flavour and extra nourishment by using culinary herbs, balsamic vinegar, sun-dried tomatoes, garlic and ginger.
- Be sensible about fat intake but don't cut it out altogether. Fat isn't all bad. As well as providing vita-mins and essential fatty acids, it satiates hunger and reduces the temptation to snack on junk. However, feel free to snack on healthier items. Any kind of fresh

fruit is good. Or how about a bowl of home-made vegetable soup, a green salad, half an avocado with oil and vinegar dressing, sticks of raw veg with curd cheese or soda bread with a little butter and real honey? Research shows that eating little and often not only improves digestion but helps to keep kilos and cholesterol in check!

- Promise yourself that you'll eat plenty of fresh fruit as between-meal snacks. This improves vitamin and mineral intake and, at the same time, cancels cravings. Keeping blood glucose well balanced in this way is great for preventing mid-morning binges and mid-afternoon slumps in energy.

- Don't deep-fry anything, and avoid take-aways and pre-packaged foods that are high in fat. Say no to yellow spreads (and any other foods) that are made with hydrogenated vegetable oils. Foods that provide natural polyunsaturates – from seeds, nuts, vegetables and cold-pressed oils – are particularly important. Use extra-virgin olive oil for cooking and a little butter or non-hydrogenated margarine for spreading.

- If cheese, cream, mayonnaise, ice-cream or yoghurt are on your regular shopping list and you usually choose low-fat varieties, go instead for the full-fat versions and eat half the quantity that you would normally. Low-fat equivalents are often loaded with artificial additives (yet more toxins) which, some experts believe, can cause weight increase by encouraging liver toxicity.

- Go for heaps of wholegrains, fresh vegetables and salads, fresh and canned fish, organic poultry (minus the skin), free-range eggs, soya beans, beancurd, lentils, seeds, chickpeas, organic jacket potatoes, fresh and dried fruit, real cheeses and live yoghurt made from sheep's or goat's milk. Swap white rice for brown. Up your intake of pasta: if you want to increase variety, health stores have a huge range of tasty non-wheat alternatives to ordinary spaghetti, made from rice, buckwheat and rye – quick to cook and well worth trying.

- Avoid ordinary sandwich bread – the spongy stuff that lasts for days. It is made from mass-produced bread wheat and usually laced heavily with extra yeast and extra gluten (both common allergens) and dosed with a number of additives. Sensitivity to wheat-based foods can be the sole cause of some weight problems! Good alternatives are yeast-free soda bread (check the label, some soda bread isn't yeast-free), rye bread or pumpernickel (black rye). Brown pitta bread does contain yeast but less of it and may still be a better option than a standard loaf that's loaded with additives. It's worth remembering that the denser the texture the better the bread, and these are the foods that help most to satiate your appetite, provide improved levels of nourishment and reduce the risk of binges and cravings.

- Start the day with a decent meal and don't be tempted to miss meals during the day. It won't help weight problems in the long term.

- If you have a tendency to overeat, try dishing meals up on smaller plates. Quantities still look generous but you'll avoid bingeing.

- Get up and go! Introduce two teaspoons of organic linseeds or a teaspoon of Linoforce granules into your daily routine. These gentle forms of fibre encourage a sluggish bowel into life and can help to get rid of clogged wastes.

- I know I've said it before but it really does make a difference to weight and energy levels if you sit down to meals. Take a few moments to calm yourself before tucking in. Breathe more deeply. Chew everything thoroughly and rest for ten minutes after the last mouthful. These are simple but effective ways of improving the chances of food being utilized properly.

- Don't allow mealtimes to be disrupted by the demands of other people. If someone wants something while you are eating, suggest calmly that they wait until you have finished. You're not a slave. You owe it to yourself to enjoy your own food and to nourish yourself.

- Avoid colours such as red, orange and yellow in plates, tableware, napkins or cutlery. The reason so many fast-food outlets make use of these colours is because they know it encourages you to eat more! Instead, go for green, turquoise or light blue. If necessary, change the paint in your dining area and kitchen, and avoid wearing reds and oranges too.

- Take more exercise. Apart from helping to strengthen bones, tone muscles and reduce the risk of heart disease, exercise also stimulates the body to shed toxins. A 20–30-minute brisk walk each day (40 to 60 minutes three times a week) encourages a balanced appetite. If your lifestyle really doesn't allow time to exercise outside, consider the possibility of having exercise equipment at home. Could you find space in the spare room, garage or shed for a treadmill, rowing machine, stationary bike or rebounder (mini-trampoline)? Rebounding is a great way to improve lymph drainage and provides good exercise without jarring the spine or joints.

- Remember, where weight problems have not responded to any other type of diet, an increasing number of practitioners now recommend a programme of food combining. Try it initially for 30 days and then for, say, four or five days a week to maintain a sensible balance. Do keep in mind that food combining does not involve calorie-counting or portion-weighing.

- If nothing you do makes any difference, I would very strongly recommend a consultation with a qualified nutrition practitioner. Intractable weight problems can be caused by conditions such as candidiasis and hypoglycaemia, both of which respond well to nutritional treatment. The Directory on page 139 will tell you how to find help.

Simply Food Combining

❧

❧

We are living in a great age, and never before was
the desirability, not to say the necessity, for good
health in more urgent need.

Dr William Howard Hay, 1934

Food combining has many dedicated followers. Among
them are those who suffered for many years with apparently intractable illnesses that had never responded to
drugs or surgery but found that food combining 'fixed it'.
Thousands of others have discovered that food combining
is the only form of eating that deals safely and permanently
with excess weight.

It is estimated that around half the population – one in every two people – don't digest their food well enough or absorb enough nourishment to maintain ideal health and energy levels. A frightening statistic. Food combining can help here, too, by improving the way the body digests food. And it's particularly effective at settling bowel disorders such as constipation and irritable bowel syndrome (IBS).

A Long and Prestigious History

Food combining was first recorded by ancient tribes, called Essenes, in Palestine around 2000 years ago. The first 'modern' medical interest came from a group of American doctors, called Natural Hygienists, back in the 1860s. More studies were carried out towards the end of the nineteenth century and beginning of the twentieth century which substantiated earlier findings that, when the body does not digest food properly, the resulting toxic overload can lead to disease.

Probably the most useful and important in-depth research occurred from the mid-1920s until the early 1980s. Dr Herbert Shelton, considered by many practitioners to be the leading researcher into food combining as we know it today, spent almost 60 years compiling data on how different food combinations affect body processes. He wrote several highly regarded books and papers on the subject.

Although food combining is sometimes known as 'The Hay Diet' because of its association with Dr William Howard Hay, he didn't invent the system. In fact, Dr Hay's ideas tended to be more complicated – and differ considerably – from earlier research and from the much simpler form of food combining that I now recommend. This is not to say that his methods did not work. On the contrary, many people have benefited greatly from his advice and his writings. However, if you have not tried food combining before, or have been put off by too many rules and regulations, you should find the tips in this chapter refreshingly easy to follow.

So What is Food Combining?

A healthy-eating programme based on the simple principle of not mixing proteins and starches at the same meal. Although a better title might be 'Food Separation', it does not mean that food combiners eat everything entirely separately; rather that they choose to enjoy their food in slightly different combinations.

Proteins

In food-combining terms, the only proteins we need to concern ourselves with are those listed on page 56, which include meat, poultry, cheese, fish and eggs.

Starches

For the purposes of food combining, starches include cereals, biscuits, bread and potatoes. A full list appears on page 57.

This Goes With That

The most important food-combining maxim is that proteins are not mixed with starches, but you'll find a whole list of versatile vegetables and salad foods on pages 56–57 that will happily mix with both.

BUT SURELY STARCH AND PROTEIN TURN UP TOGETHER IN ALL KINDS OF FOOD?

A very long list of foods contain both protein and starch. In fact, almost every food you could name will have a little of each. For example, cauliflower, carrots, celery, broccoli and beansprouts all include a few grams or part of a gram of both protein and starch. But these tiny quantities do not cause the digestive system any difficulty. We are concerned here only with separating those foods that contain high levels of starch or protein and which have been found, through experience or trial and error, to disagree with each other during the early stages of digestion.

How Does Food Combining Work?

Doctors who have researched the system believe that it enhances liver, kidney and bowel function and improves the way foods are digested. As a result, the body finds it easier to deal with toxicity because it is better supplied with vital vitamins and minerals and is more efficient at eliminating unwanted wastes. Food combining also plays an important role in improving and maintaining a healthy acid/alkali balance in the blood. For those interested in the science behind this, page 63 has more blurb.

Pick up any textbook on medical physiology and you'll discover that, to prepare protein foods for digestion, the stomach must produce hydrochloric acid. But starchy foods fare better without being swamped by stomach acid – at least during the first stages of digestion. Because we commonly mix proteins and starches together – bread with cheese, chicken with potato, fish with chips – we make it more difficult for complete digestion to take place. Unfortunately, even though there may not be any noticeable symptoms of *in*digestion, it's a fact that mixed protein/starch meals are never dealt with as efficiently as those that follow food-combining guidelines.

How Does this Help to Keep the Weight Well Balanced?

If it all sounds a little strange at first, it's worth knowing that, in evolutionary terms, we've only been eating mixed meals for a relatively short time, whereas our digestive systems have not changed very much in the past ten thousand years. Aficionados agree that reducing the toxic load on the body using food-combining principles not only improves the function of all internal organs but also increases absorption and metabolism of nutrients, thereby encouraging well-balanced weight.

Here's How to Begin

- First of all, familiarize yourself with the quick reference chart on page 55 which shows you – at a glance – which foods combine well and which combinations are best avoided.
- Then, check out the PROTEIN, VEGETABLE AND STARCH suggestions on pages 56–57. These will give you lots of new shopping and menu ideas.

All you have to remember is the following formula:

1. DON'T mix any major protein food with starch at the same meal, and
2. DON'T eat fruit in the middle of – or immediately after – a main meal. Enjoy it either as a between-meal snack or as a starter – in other words, on an empty stomach. Fruit passes through the system more quickly than protein or starch and is digested more efficiently if taken without other foods.

Top Tips for Successful Combining

- Some people, when they are first introduced to food combining, imagine that they need to eat everything separately. No, it's much simpler. Say you had planned to have a
tuna or sardine salad with rice. Fish is a first-class protein. Rice is predominantly starchy. To food-combine at
this meal, all you have to do is forget the rice and serve a
larger portion of tuna or sardine with a great big salad –
OR leave out the fish and jazz up the rice by adding, for
example, sweetcorn, mixed pulses, avocado and peppers.
- Don't worry about having to food-combine every day.
If it isn't convenient, just forget it for a particular
meal. My husband Richard and I follow the system
four or five days a week and still feel the benefits.
- Eating out? If you're having chicken, lamb or fish, for
example, ask for more vegetables or salad instead of
potatoes or fries.
- Sandwiches often contain meat, egg or fish fillings –
which means that you are mixing protein and starch.
In addition, the sandwich bread itself can cause weight
problems and lethargy. Salad goes with anything and
makes an excellent filling for good bread but don't
limit yourself to the inevitable lettuce, cucumber or
tomato. Check out the Versatile Vegetables on pages
56–57 for lots of bright ideas. As an energy-lifting
alternative, why not have pasta with salad or sardines
with salad; or home-made vegetable soup with soda
bread; or fill a pitta with avocado or hummus.

- Make sure you eat enough. Don't be afraid to increase portion sizes to compensate for the fact that you are no longer mixing major proteins and starches on the same plate. Eat until you are comfortably full but not overloaded. Examples:

  You've chosen a protein-based meal so you're not including potato or other starch. Make sure that you have two eggs instead of one, or a larger fillet of fish, or a bigger breast of chicken.
  When it comes to starch-based meals and you're avoiding the protein, go up a size when you choose your jacket potato – or dish up an extra spoonful of pasta, rice or couscous.

- Once you are familiar with the basics, try to food-combine for a few days each week. This will help to reduce your intake of unwanted chemicals and enhance the benefits you are gaining from those two regular detox days!

Health department guidelines for most countries now rec-ommend that we eat five servings of fresh produce every day: two portions of green vegetables, two pieces of fresh fruit and a salad. For most people, this can be a difficult target. One of the greatest food-combining benefits is that you'll find yourself enjoying far more vegetables, salads and fruits almost without having to think about it.

At-a-glance Food Combining

Combine ANY of the foods in Column B (the centre section) with either Proteins (Column A) or Starches (Column C). But don't mix the Proteins in Column A directly with the Starches in Column C.

Column A PROTEINS	Column B MIX WITH ANYTHING	Column C STARCHES
Fish	All vegetables	Potatoes & sweet
Shellfish	except potatoes	potatoes
Free-range poultry	All salads	All grains including oats, rice, rye, couscous etc.
Free-range eggs	Salad dressings	
Lamb	Herbs & spices	All pulses except soya
Cheese	Seeds	
Yoghurt	Nuts	Biscuits
Soya	Cream	Cakes
Beef } not recommended keep these three	Maple syrup	Bread
Pork } items to a	Honey	Crackers
Milk } minimum		Pastry
	Spreading fats	
	Butter	
	Cooking oils	

Recommended PROTEIN FOODS – these will mix with any salads, vegetables (except potatoes), dressings, oils, spreading fats, seeds or nuts but not with STARCHES.

These are concentrated proteins:

Beancurd	Goat's milk cheese	Sheep's milk cheese
Buttermilk	Lamb's liver	Tofu
Free-range eggs	Lean lamb	Yoghurt (preferably
Free-range poultry	Organic cow's milk	from sheep's or
Fresh fish	Quorn	goat's milk)

I have not recommended ordinary non-organic cow's milk because it can cause digestive discomfort and seems to aggravate a number of health conditions. All major supermarkets and health-food shops stock organic milk. When it comes to yoghurt, that made from cow's milk is better tolerated than milk itself but sheep's yoghurt is better still.

VERSATILE VEGETABLE AND SALAD FOODS – THEY MIX WITH EITHER PROTEINS OR STARCHES.
Broaden your vegetable horizons. Keep this list as an all-year-round reference. Aim to eat two or three different items every day either as salad, cooked vegetables, in soups, stir-fries or casseroles:

Artichokes	Beetroot	Capsicums (red,
Asparagus	Broccoli	yellow or green
Aubergine	Brussels sprouts	bell peppers)
(Eggplant)	Cabbage (dark-	Carrots (organic
Avocado	leaf varieties	only)
Bamboo shoots	have more	Cauliflower
Beansprouts	nourishment)	Cauliflower greens
Beet greens	Calabrese	Celeriac

Recommended STARCHY FOODS – these will mix with any vegetables, salads, nuts, seeds, dressings, oils or spreading fats but not with PROTEINS.

These are concentrated starches:

Barley	Oat-based	Quinoa (say
Basmati rice	cereals	'keen-wa')
Brown rice	Oat biscuits	Rice cakes
Buckwheat grains	Oat bran	Rice flour
(Kasha)	Oats	Rye bread
Buckwheat pasta	Pasta	Rye crackers
Couscous	Pitta bread	Soda bread
Jacket potatoes	Porridge	Sweet potatoes
(organic only)	Potato flour (a useful	Wild rice
Matzo crackers	alternative to	
Muesli (choose	wheat flour)	
wheat-free or	Pumpernickel	
gluten-free)	(dark rye bread)	

Celery	Lettuce (dark-	Spring onions
Chicory	leaf varieties	Sprouted seeds
Chives	have more	Sugarsnap peas
Courgette	nourishment)	Swede (rutabaga)
(zucchini)	Mangetout	Tomatoes
Culinary herbs	Marrow	Turnip greens
Dandelion greens	Mushrooms	Turnips
Eggplant	Mustard & cress	Watercress
(Aubergine)	Onion	Zucchini
Endive	Purple sprouting	(courgette)
Garlic	Rutabaga (swede)	
Kale	Shallots	
Leek	Spinach	

Healthy Snack Suggestions

If you are stuck for snack ideas, here are a few suggestions for healthy snacks which follow food-combining guidelines.

- A bowl of home-made vegetable soup
- A pot of fresh sheep's milk yoghurt stirred with a teaspoon of best quality honey and a sprinkling of flaked almonds. (Sheep's milk yoghurt is available from all major supermarkets; cold-pressed honey at good health-food shops.)
- Any kind of fresh fruit
- Half a dozen dried figs with a handful of unblanched almonds
- Corn chips (additive-free, from a health store) dunked into aubergine dip
- Half an avocado pear with olive oil and balsamic vinegar dressing
- Hummus on rice cakes or rye crackers
- A couple of small organic potatoes, washed and sliced with the skins on. Sauté them in a little extra-virgin olive oil until tender and beginning to brown and serve with buttered Naan bread
- Sticks of raw vegetables (crudités) with curd cheese
- Yeast-free soda bread or Matzo crackers spread with a little butter and cold-pressed honey
- If you're travelling or have no choice but to miss a meal, mix a handful of any of these in any combination to make a satisfying snack:

Pumpkin seeds	Sunflower seeds
Pine nuts	Walnuts
Brazils	Unblanched almonds
Macadamia nuts	Hazelnuts
Flaked almonds	Pecans

Organic dried fruit, especially dried figs

Kathryn Marsden's Swap Sheet

Whether you food-combine or not, you're more likely to maintain better digestion and elimination (and balanced bodyweight) by eating fewer of the items in COLUMN A and more of those in COLUMN B.

COLUMN A	COLUMN B
Deep-fried food	Grill, bake, casserole, steam, stir-fry or wok it instead
Cooking oils	Extra-virgin olive oil
Margarine or low-fat spreads	Butter or non-hydrogenated spread
Crisps and peanuts	Almonds, brazils, hazelnuts, macadamias, pecans, walnuts, sunflower seeds, pumpkin seeds
Sweets and cakes	Wholegrain cereal bars, natural liquorice, dried fruits, fresh fruit
Chocolate	Green & Black Organic chocolate (it's delicious)
Packaged orange juice	Apple or grape juice, or buy a juicer and make your own
Coffee, tea and cola	Savoury beverages, water, fresh fruit juice, vegetable juice, herbal fruit teas, soup.
Battery or barn-raised poultry & eggs	Organic free-range poultry & eggs
Wheat-based or sugar-coated cereal	Oat porridge, gluten-free (wheat-free) muesli
Cow's milk	Soya milk, oat milk, almond milk or Rice Dream
Cow's milk cheeses	Sheep's or goat's cheeses

Ordinary mass-produced bread	Yeast-free soda bread, pumpernickel, rye, rice cakes, oat cakes, oat biscuits, Matzos, pittas
Beef or pork	Fresh fish (especially the oily kinds such as sardine, mackerel, wild salmon and trout), lean lamb, lamb's liver, organic free-range poultry
Convenience meals and take-aways	Prepare more of your own from fresh basic ingredients so that you know what goes into them
Foods full of additives	Food that aren't!

AUTHOR'S NOTE: Food combining is now recommended by an increasing number of practitioners to their patients. However, like detoxification, the method has one or two determined detractors who say that the idea of eating proteins separately from starches is nonsense (a good word, apparently, if you don't really know what you're talking about but want to sound authoritative). I asked one critic, a dietitian, who was adamant that food combining has no basis in fact, if she had any evidence that it didn't work or that it had caused any unpleasant side effects. She replied that she 'couldn't say' because she had 'never tried it'. She just knew it wasn't effective.

Everyone is, of course, entitled to their own opinion.

I leave the following words to speak for themselves:

'It is impossible to believe that the opponents from seats of learning know anything about the effects of diet. Wounded vanity makes them hurl their high-brow articles against new science into the newspapers ... an act which, from the standpoint of general welfare, can only be considered arrogant.' Penned in 1934, these are the words of Dr Max Bircher-Benner, considered by his peers to be 'a born physician, counted among the great ones in the history of medicine'.

Dealing with Over-Acidity –
The Importance of Balancing
Blood Chemistry

ॐ

ACID-FORMING AND ALKALINE-FORMING
FOODS – KNOW THE DIFFERENCE – HELP
FOR CRAVINGS AND ALLERGIES

ॐ

Substances to neutralize acidity, to absorb gas, to relieve pain and gastric irritation are employed by the trainload to aid the digestion of food. Millions of dollars are spent yearly for drugs which afford a temporary respite from the discomfort and distress that result from the decomposition of food in the stomach and the intestine.

Dr Herbert M. Shelton

Maintenance of good health depends upon many factors. One of the most important is a precisely balanced internal chemistry that makes sure our blood is neither too acid nor too alkaline.

This can sound complicated.

It doesn't have to be.

Regular cleansing, especially when used in conjunction with a food-combining diet, is one of the best ways to ensure an optimum acid/alkali balance.

A number of health books include elaborate explanations of the need for such balance, to the point where the reader is utterly confused. Even now, I receive mail from people who, labouring over the terminology, have struggled to fathom some unnecessarily involved procedures, worrying that they are making some unforgivable mistake by not including the right foods in the right quantities. In order to follow the *Food Combining 2-Day Detox*, it simply is not necessary to get bogged down with garbled gobbledegook.

However, keeping our blood supply shipshape is crucial to maintaining good health in general. So, if you'd like to know how and why, stick with me here. Otherwise, skip to the next section on page 66.

Is It Acid or Alkali?

To gauge whether something is acid or alkali, scientists use a scale of numbers and a measurement called *pH*. Anything that is strongly acidic attracts a low number: stomach acid, for example, has a *pH* of 1.1. Alkalis attract higher numbers: bicarbonate of soda measures a *pH* of 12. In other words, when the numbers go up, the acidity goes down and vice versa. Water is neither acid nor alkaline and is given a *pH* of 7, meaning neutral. Thus, anything under 7 is considered acid; anything over 7 is seen as alkaline.

Still with me?
It gets simpler!

The most likely place that we will have seen these two letters – '*pH*' – is on skin-care products. Skin secretions are slightly acid, measuring a *pH* that varies between 5.0 and 5.6. When we buy cleansers, toners or moisturizers, the label will sometimes tell us that the product is *pH balanced*; in other words, designed to 'match' our skin's natural *pH*. The idea behind this thinking is that, by pitching the product *pH* to the skin's own *pH*, the natural protective covering of the skin's surface (called the acid mantle) is less likely to be disturbed. Specialists know that when skin pH is damaged, skin becomes more open to infections, dryness or oiliness and may age more quickly; *pH-balanced* products aim to reduce this risk. One reason why ordinary soap is not always an ideal cleanser is because it is very alkaline and disturbs the skin's defences. Skin *pH* will also be affected by the efficiency (or otherwise) of your digestion and your nutritional status.

Stomach acid	Wine	Skin	Water	Blood	Sea Water	Bicarbonate of soda	Caustic Soda	
1.1	3.5	5.0–5.6	7.0	7.45/6	8.1	12.0	14.0	pH

Blood is only slightly alkaline at 7.45/7.46. Any great differences can lead very quickly to serious illness and death. For example, 6.9 can cause diabetic coma whereas 7.7 may result in convulsions. When considering ideal levels, some experts see 7.4 as too acid and 7.5 as far too alkaline, sufficiently irregular, they say, to cause concern. Even the tiniest variations can make the difference between feeling great or feeling grouchy. Happily, the body has several control mechanisms available to maintain a fairly steady *pH*. Special buffering systems call upon reserves from mineral stores in bone and blood to correct the balance. However, these will only move into gear if the body is adequately supplied with those minerals in the first place.

Although it is possible to achieve an over-alkaline system (for example, by eating too many vegetables and fruits but not enough protein or starch), for most of us the opposite is the case. Blood is usually too acid. To make sure that the body is in a position to neutralize an over-acid system, we need to increase our intake of alkalizing (sometimes referred to as *alkaline-forming*) foods. They cushion the corrosive effects of too much acid in the bloodstream, help to repair and rebuild cells, and cleanse and invigorate the blood and tissues.

It works like this: Foods are classified not by how acid or alkaline they are *before* they are swallowed but by what effect they have on the body *after* digestion. Many foods that *taste* acidic (grapes, lemons) are, in fact, *alkaline-forming* foods because, after metabolism, they leave behind an alkalizing ash deposit of minerals (such as calcium, magnesium, potassium or iron) that help to 'mop up' surplus acid. On the other hand, most of the bland foods (meat, fish, eggs, and most cereals) are acid-forming in that they deposit acid ash of sulphur, phosphorous or chlorine, making an acid system even more acid. When we eat more alkaline-forming foods, we help to rid the body of excess phosphoric, sulphuric and uric acids.

This can be particularly helpful to anyone who is trying to deal with any kind of addiction, such as alcohol, cigarettes, sugar. Reducing acid overload reduces cravings. It has also helped relieve the misery of premenstrual 'waterlogging'.

Improving the acid/alkali ratio has shown an excellent response in patients with hay fever, other allergies and asthma. This may be because of the way alkaline-forming foods help to detoxify the blood and encourage the liver to function more efficiently.

When the liver is under pressure (see page 73), digestion is sluggish and natural food substances that are normally dealt with easily and innocuously can begin to cause sensitivity. Partially digested foods trigger an increase in the production of histamine, the hormonal messenger which is produced in response to an allergen. A toxic or stressed liver may not be able to efficiently detoxify histamine which then builds up in the system, initiating further allergic reactions. Ironically, overuse of antihistamine medication can inhibit the liver's ability to clear excess histamine away from the body.

Acid-forming Foods are Good for Us, Too!

Although by increasing our intake of vegetables, salads and fruits, and cutting back a little on the heavier stodge, we can help the body to neutralize excess acidity, that doesn't mean we should eat only alkalizing foods and ignore the acid-forming foods. Acid and alkaline ash perform different vital functions. To maintain an ideal balance, we need to eat both. However, many people have a tendency to overdo the acid-forming bread, the pizza or the sugary 'treats', and to bypass the alkalizing vegetables. Meat, gravy and sweet desserts, without which most men's lives would end, are all very acid-forming. However, other acid-formers, such as oily fish, cheese, eggs, poultry and soya, are nourishing and should be part of a healthily balanced diet.

Sour Face?

And, yes, in case you're wondering, there is a connection between an acid system and an acrid attitude. A caustic, churlish, disagreeable or grudging personality may have many reasons for being out of sorts with the world but can sometimes be linked to fussy eating habits, a dislike of fruit, an aversion to vegetables and insistence that meat is essential at every meal. A grey pallor, oily or dull hair, sour breath and any persistently unpleasant body smells are all signs of an over-acid system. So, too, are poor digestion, headaches and constipation.

Watch out for types who poke food about their plates as if they were operating on it, or refer to 'foreign stuff', or make rhetorical remarks such as 'This is vegetarian, isn't it?'

Health problems that might be aggravated, or perhaps even triggered, by over-acidity include:

Arthritis	Lethargy
Diabetes	Muscle pain
Gout	Osteoporosis
Kidney problems	Poor lung function

> There are other aspects of our lives, apart from diet, that contribute to an over-acid system. Smoking, stress, late nights, fear, worry, anxiety and excess alcohol are good examples. Poor blood flow to the tissues causes acid accumulation so anything that improves circulation, such as regular exercise, is alkalizing. So, too, is deeper breathing, because it increases the supply of oxygen and other nutrients around the body and chases out more carbon dioxide waste.

You'll be pleased to know that it isn't necessary to remember long lists of which foods are alkaline-forming and which are acid-forming. The food-combining format, especially if used in conjunction with regular 2-day cleansing, automatically provides a natural balance of the right levels of each type. However, it does help to keep in mind that:

Foods that take longer to digest (meat, fish, cereals, beans) are more likely to be acid-forming. They include:

Bread	Fish & shellfish
Cereals: oats, rice, wheat	Meat
Cheese	Pasteurized milk
Eggs	Poultry

Foods that pass more quickly through the system (fruit, vegetables and salads) tend to be alkalizing:

All kinds of seeds including sunflower, pumpkin, poppy and sesame

All salad foods

Almonds

Brazils

Fresh and frozen vegetables Just to be contrary, asparagus, most pulses and olives are acid-forming. However, they are still extremely good for you!

Fresh fruit

Live yoghurt

Buttermilk

Dried fruit

Fresh and dried herbs

Whey

Anyone wanting to know more about acid/alkali balance in relation to food intake is recommended to read:
Food and Healing by Annemarie Colbin (Ballantine Books)
The Wright Diet by Celia Wright (Green Library)
The Whole Health Manual by Patrick Holford (Thorsons)
Food Combining In 30 Days or *The Food Combining Diet* both by Kathryn Marsden (Thorsons)

Looking After Your Liver

჻

჻

LIVER, n. *A large red organ thoughtfully provided by
nature to be bilious with.*

Ambrose Bierce {1842–1914}

Our familiar greeting of 'How are you?' translates in some
countries of the world as 'How is your liver today?' In
Chinese medicine, the health of the liver and gallbladder
is seen to have a profound effect upon our openness and
receptivity to people and ideas. We talk in terms of
a person having an 'open' personality or being open-
minded. The opposite would be someone who is bigoted,
dogmatic and uncompromising – someone who, according
to Oriental doctors, might be troubled with liver problems
too.

Physiologically, the liver is a complex organ which carries out an amazing number of different jobs:

It takes proteins from the food we eat, breaks them down and builds them up again into entirely different structures (a bit like Lego) that are then used for a wide variety of tasks including body repairs and rebuilding.

It is a store cupboard for energy-producing starches, fats and sugars and for some vitamins and minerals.

Without the liver, we wouldn't be able to digest fats.

How does it do that?

The liver produces a couple of pints of bile each day.

Don't like the sound of it?

You should know how incredibly important it is to helping keep the body detoxified. When bile doesn't flow freely, toxins build up, poisons are not released and the resulting congestion can lead to liver damage and serious ill health.

Bile is stored in a sac below the liver called the gallbladder and squeezed out into the small intestine when we eat any meal that contains fat. The bile salts then help digest fatty substances and assist in the absorption of some micronutrients.

The liver is a major blood reservoir, filtering around two pints of blood every minute! In that blood are vital foods – plus a number of unwanted substances. The liver is in charge of filtering, transforming and discharging the 'not-so-desirables' that are collected from food, water, medication and environmental pollutants, as well as those produced within the body as a result of internal processes. Bile flow is one way in which the liver gets rid of a variety of chemical compounds including unwanted hormone residues, drugs and pesticides.

No wonder this amazing organ gets tired!

At one time or another, almost everyone is bound to have felt 'liverish'. There's nothing abnormal about being a bit 'under the weather' – occasionally! However, because the liver is so closely involved in so many metabolic processes, even minor sluggishness can have profound effects on energy levels and general wellbeing. Being kind to the liver and giving it all the help it needs is therefore absolutely essential to the success of any detoxification programme. Long-term care can help protect it from further damage and may also provide additional unexpected health benefits. There are encouraging reports of liver cleansing reducing asthma attacks, lowering cholesterol, enhancing thyroid function, lifting the misery of premenstrual tension, clearing eczema and psoriasis and helping solve stubborn weight problems by speeding metabolism.

A sensation of tightness around the chest and upper abdomen

Distended abdomen

Coated tongue

Sour taste in the mouth, especially first thing in the morning

Easy bruising or web-shaped red spots on the skin

Eye problems including night blindness

Yellowing of the whites of the eyes

Dark circles around the eyes

Difficulty digesting fatty food

Nausea

Vertigo or dizziness

Persistent headaches

Yellow or mucusy stools

Mucus in the throat or nose

Sinus problems

Food sensitivities, especially to wheat products or fats

Depression

Hyper-excitability

Irrational anger

Bilious temperament

One or two of these symptoms in isolation do not necessarily indicate liver problems. However, anyone who identifies more than three or four of those listed might benefit from seeing a qualified nutrition practitioner or medical herbalist for further investigation.

Liver Nourishment

You won't be surprised if I tell you that a diet rich in saturated or chemically altered fats, alcohol or sugar is not recommended. One that is high in the right kind of dietary fibre and contains plenty of antioxidant-rich plant foods *definitely is* – because it encourages optimum liver function, helping to increase bile flow and to guard cells from free-radical damage.

Free radicals are highly reactive molecules that can destroy cells and initiate degeneration and disease. Antioxidant nutrients such as vitamins A, C, B6, E, beta-carotene, selenium and zinc are able to scavenge free radicals and prevent oxidative damage.

The foods and other factors recommended in this detoxification and after-care programme are designed to give the liver the best kind of support possible.

Resilient Liver

It is astonishing that the liver survives so well in spite of the constant onslaught of toxic chemicals. The effects of the current levels of exposure that we all face have yet to be determined but concerned health experts believe that we are already witnessing a marked increase in a whole range of diseases as a direct result of untreated chemical toxicity.

The Liver and our Emotions

Ask almost anyone which part of the body is responsible for controlling the emotions and the answer will almost certainly be the brain. The liver has many diverse functions all essential to life, including the vital processing, detoxification and removal of foreign poisons – all obviously physical and physiological. But the idea that liver imbalances can also affect our innermost feelings is not well known. It is certainly not accepted as a sound theory by general medicine. And yet, just look at some of the words that we use in common language to describe both physical and emotional distress:

Liverish is a word used to describe that feeling of being 'off colour', 'queasy' or 'bilious'. But it can also mean disagreeable, ill-humoured, crusty and irritable.

Choleric, medically, means 'causing biliousness', but emotionally describes annoyance and exasperation.

Gall (the old name for bile) is a bitter substance. The word 'gall' can be taken to mean brass nerve and impertinence as in 'the gall of the fellow' but also equates with anger, outrage and insult.

And then there is *Bitterness*, a useless, time-wasting and empty emotion. Bile is 'bitter as any gall', of course. And although it doesn't follow in every case, there is some evidence that, where there is any problem with bile flow or gallbladder disease, there can be an underlying bitterness in the person. The patient may not acknowledge its existence but can still harbour hostility or resentment over present or past relationships, actions or mistakes. Where bile flow is blocked – by gallstones, for example – there can be blocked aggression. Some observers suggest that not expressing real feelings for fear of upsetting someone, 'biting one's tongue', the need to 'keep the peace' and the reluctance or inability to 'have a go' at someone may explain why gallstones appear more frequently in married women than in single women or in men. This 'pleaser syndrome' also applies in liver disease.

Jaundiced people may be bitter as well as bigoted, envious, jealous and prejudiced. These emotions are not always apparent on the surface of someone's personality but may lurk in the subconscious. The condition of jaundice is caused when the yellow bile pigment called bilirubin is trapped in congested bile. Instead of being released through the intestines, it is reabsorbed through the bloodstream, causing a yellowing of the skin and the whites of the eyes. Bilirubin is made from old red blood cells and is the natural colouring of faeces, in case you're interested.

The Mind/Body Connection

Most medical doctors consider the mind and the body to be totally separate entities, and treat mental and physical illness accordingly. Even those who acknowledge that stubbornness of will can help to bring about remission of illness are reluctant to accept that physical manifestation of disease could ever have been actually *caused* by a sad spirit, an undermined personality or eroded self-esteem. On the other hand, experts who treat the psychological aspects of illness are more likely to see an emotional or mental angle attached to most physical maladies.

Researchers studying the relatively new mind/body science of psycho-neuro-immunology (PNI) can demonstrate clearly what many have known for years – that the mind has greater control over body function and health than does the body directly. There is a sentence somewhere among the essays of Plutarch, the Greek biographer, which tells us that if the body should ever take the mind to court and sue it for damages, '*it would be found that the mind had been a ruinous tenant to its landlord*'. Nowhere is this more graphically illustrated than in disorders of the digestion, liver and bowel.

If liver function is failing, the liver becomes unable to evaluate and distinguish between what should be stored and what needs to be excreted, and this allows poisons to accumulate. In the mind, this may translate as indecisiveness, an inability to assess situations or tell the difference between acceptable and unacceptable actions or behaviour.

The liver stores and generates energy. On an emotional level it can store good positive energy but also negative energy, the most damaging being that of suppressed anger. Hoarding rage and resentment can lead to loss of vitality as well as digestive disturbance. When the 'toxins of anger' accumulate, then the toxins in our diet only add to the disharmony that already exists in the liver.

Coping and Changing

Physically applied therapies such as diet, herbal medicine, reflexology, massage and colonic irrigation have all been shown to bring excellent improvements in such conditions. However, good companionship, music, rest and relaxation, a sensible level of exercise, proper sleep and the right mental attitude are all just as important and fundamental to complete recovery and long-term wellbeing.

People Pressure

It's well known that stress, anxiety and emotional pain can cause and contribute to many diseases. But, sometimes, it can be more a case of *who* is wrong with you rather than *what* is wrong with you. It's an unavoidable fact of life that, sometimes, there are other people who are not good for your health. They can invade your inner space, eat away at your resolve, blackmail your emotions and destroy your self-esteem. Learning to deal with difficult relationships, either by ending them or by protecting yourself from them, is fundamental to the success of any health programme.

If a condition is not responding to treatment despite all that is being tried, I believe it is very much worthwhile investigating, with honesty, the possibility that some problem of the mind may be holding back physical recovery. Past experiences and childhood hurts, dark corners at the back of the memory bank, are the best places to begin.

Talking really does help. Have you ever noticed that when we are close to a problem that has been bugging us for sometime, our perspective gets lost? Insignificant things become deadly serious. Molehills turn into mountains. Dreams become nightmares. Talking to an independent someone, outside the problem relationship, is a first step to shedding any emotional load. The old adage of a trouble shared being a trouble halved really does hold true. An unclouded second opinion can be very helpful. Asking for help is not a sign of weakness but of strength.

Help from Herbal Medicines

On the basis that prevention is always preferable to cure – and in addition to eating lots of foods rich in antioxidants and taking a daily antioxidant supplement – it makes good health sense to treat the liver to an occasional herbal clean-up. The detox part of the *Food Combining 2-Day Detox* is designed to take the strain off the liver, encourage elimination of stockpiled poisons and replenish the body's depleted stores of nourishment.

In conjunction with the food side of the *Food Combining 2-Day Detox*, follow a course of liver-cleansing herbs (see page 80). I have seen some quite remarkable results following the use of herbal treatments.

Dandelion (*Taraxacum officinale*) is so nutritious that you wonder why it is left to roadsides and rabbits. It is particularly rich in vitamins, minerals, proteins, pectins, choline and carotenoids, all loved by the liver. Studies have proved that dandelion is one of the finest liver remedies, clearing congestion, improving bile flow and reducing inflammation. The leaves and the root have been used to help patients with gallstones and jaundice. Dandelion is also used as a major ingredient in a number of proprietary branded herbal medicines. Weight for weight, dandelion leaves contain 25 per cent more beta-carotene than carrots. The leaves make a wonderful salad vegetable and yet this far-from-humble weed is rarely used. Freshly picked, well-washed and finely chopped young leaves can give a boring salad a real lift. Don't pick them from anywhere near kerbs or hedgerows where traffic passes by or where you suspect they may have been sprayed with weedkiller.

Milk Thistle (*Silybum marianum*), not to be confused with the common thistle, protects the liver in several different ways. Apart from being a powerful antioxidant, it has been shown to have a positive effect in serious conditions such as cirrhosis, hepatitis, alcohol-induced damage and in inflammation of the bile duct. Milk thistle also protects against a range of extremely dangerous toxic chemicals.

Artichoke (*Cynara scolymus*) has a long and prestigious history in the treatment of many types of liver disease. Like dandelion and milk thistle, the leaves are used by modern medical herbalists when treating liver congestion and toxicity. Artichoke is also well known for its regenerating and protective effects and has been shown in studies to help lower blood fats and cholesterol. It's healthy and good to eat too.

If you decide to give herbal medicines a try, stick to ready-prepared branded capsules, tablets or tinctures. Use loose medicinal herbs only under the guidance of a fully quali-fied medical herbalist. Likewise, herbal medicines are not suitable for young children unless prescribed by a qualified practitioner following a test for liver function.

Highly Recommended

The herbs mentioned above can help to enhance the effects of the food-combining and detox programmes. If several of the symptoms mentioned sound like you, I believe it can really be worthwhile following a course of liver and gallbladder herbs. I have found the best results by taking a two month course either of Bioforce Boldocynara (also labelled Cynarasan in some countries) or Biocare Silymarin Complex. Details are on pages 140–41.

Colon Cleansing –
Curative or Cranky?

~

Health is not valued till sickness comes.

Proverb

Colon cleansing is a fundamental part of any detoxification programme. And if the amount of clutter we carry around in our colons is anything to go by, it could be a good idea. Astonishing as it may seem, it's estimated that most of us are weighed down by four to five pounds of stagnant and static waste – and that's in addition to what we pass each day. In some cases, especially in the chronically consti- pated and in the elderly, a backlog of twenty-five pounds of gunge is, apparently, not unusual.

If you wonder why the debris doesn't flow naturally away, it's because it has formed itself firmly into the pockets that make up the colon wall – stuck fast, a bit like black superglue, or, as one American doctor describes it, 'the consistency of truck-tire rubber'. If allowed to remain, the bowel wall becomes inaccessible to passing nutrients and fluids. And because the population of friendly flora in the gut is reduced or destroyed, the natural defences are depleted. Unfriendly bacteria and toxins are able to penetrate the wall and be reabsorbed into the bloodstream. The result is a condition called autointoxication. The word has nothing to do with being drunk and disorderly but indicates polluted blood and toxic tissues. Lethargy, lack of energy and general malaise are often the first signs of a silted and sluggish bowel.

Naturopathic medicine practitioners believe that many serious diseases begin in the bowel, long before more severe or identifiable symptoms become apparent. Improving function and speeding elimination not only relieves – or, in some cases, clears completely – existing bowel problems but can also act as a prevention against future illness.

But there are still those who disagree. For example, one grey-faced and anally retentive medic sallies blindly and fairly frequently forth with the uninformed and unintelligent sweeping statement 'bowel cleansing is a complete nonsense' (Whoops! It's nonsense again!). And yet he looks as though he himself would benefit from a *lengthy* course of colonic irrigation.

Anyone who doubts the need to improve colonic health should study the findings of the British surgeon Sir Arbuthnot Lane or the American researcher Dr Bernard Jensen. The intrepid Dr Jensen documented many case histories throughout his career, cataloguing the improvements in each condition as treatment progressed. What is most impressive is that he even took the trouble to photograph and weigh the wastes that exuded from patients who followed his cleansing diet programme. Dr

Jensen records that one particular patient discharged three gallons of hard toxic material after just one treatment.

A study carried out in 1981 by medical researchers at the University of San Francisco showed that toxic substances produced by the bowel can have a profound effect on the health of other parts of the body and may increase the risk of developing cancer, not only of the bowel but also of the breast. In a study of nearly 1500 women, it was found that those who were severely constipated and emptied their bowels less than three times a week had abnormal cells in the fluid extracted from their breast tissue. These abnormalities occurred five times as often as in those women who had daily bowel movements.

One of the greatest benefits of the *Food Combining 2-Day Detox* is that it encourages healthier bowel function. If food-combining principles are also followed in between occasional detox sessions, it is not unusual to expect two or even three daily bowel movements, one for each main meal. As a result, waste matter is released regularly from the intestines and does not get the chance to toxify the blood.

There are several ways of releasing very resistant pockets of waste. One is to swallow a course of special fibre and herbs that gently ease away the build-up and excrete it safely. Fibre and herb products can be used as a separate treatment or in conjunction with colonic irrigation.

Oral colon-cleansing products are usually based on psyllium husk fibre, pectin, herbs, probiotics (friendly gut flora) and, sometimes, linseeds, which are an excellent source of both soluble and insoluble fibre. Together, they help to rid the pockets of the large intestine of accumulated matter, encourage a lazy bowel back to life and reinstate beneficial flora. They also assist in cleansing the blood and enhancing liver and kidney function and lymph drainage.

If you decide to try using psyllium husks, linseeds or other sources of fibre that may be unfamiliar to you or that you haven't tried before, it is better to begin at a very low dose (say, two capsules or a teaspoon only per day) for three or four days. Make absolutely sure that you add extra fluid to your daily intake and then increase the fibre gradually to the quantity recommended on the pack.

Good products include: Biocare Colon Cleansing Capsules, Bioforce Linoforce, Linusit Gold Organic Linseeds, Natural Flow Psyllium Husks and Regular Ten Fibre Supplement. Stockist details are on page 139.

Colonic Irrigation

The other method of cleaning out the colon is to hose it out from below. Colonic irrigation is recommended to anyone suffering from Chronic Fatigue Syndrome (ME), yeast overgrowth, arthritis, psoriasis, eczema, acne, diverticular disease, and also in more serious cases of constipation and colonic impaction. I understand that it has worked well for those with irritable bowel syndrome (IBS).

However, I have found that removal of common allergens from the diet and the introduction of food combining are also effective for this condition. Colonic irrigation is unlikely to be sufficient on its own. Responsible therapists will guide their clients towards healthier eating, increased fluid consumption (especially fresh vegetable juices) and regular exercise. Without these improvements, your inner tubes will soon go back to being foul and fouled up.

So what does a bowel wash-out involve? Even if they have never experienced a treatment, most people have heard of colonic irrigation. Never one to recommend anything that I haven't tried, I've notched up two colonics – so I know the ropes, so to speak.

When you arrive for your appointment, you will be asked to remove undergarments, put on a gown and lie on your side on the couch. Two small disposable tubes are connected to a lubricated nozzle which is then inserted only an inch and a bit into the anus (back passage). Warm filtered water, pumped into the colon through one of the tubes, then passes the length of the large intestine. The water helps to soften and dislodge debris which then comes back, with the now soiled water, and is disposed of through the second tube. Treatment takes from 45 minutes to an hour and most people are recommended to have between two and six treatments. That's because old faecal matter sticks in the pockets of the colon wall and will not pass out naturally without some encouragement! I know a few enthusiasts who make regular six-monthly appointments as part of a long-term general health-care package.

Let's look at the pros and cons:

- Colonic irrigation is seen by a number of medics as an unnatural and potentially hazardous practice which, in unskilled hands, could cause perforation of the bowel. The only area where they acknowledge it might be useful is in an elderly person with severe compaction.

  To practice colonic therapy requires comprehensive training and is usually only offered to medically qualified practitioners or health professionals with a minimum of two years' practice experience in an alternative therapy. They all have full professional indemnity insurance and are bound by strict disciplinary codes of practice. It is therefore unlikely that anyone would find themselves 'in unskilled hands'. However, it is wise to approach a recognised organization to find a suitable therapist. Page 148 has details.

- Colonic cleansing encourages eating disorders.

  It is most certainly true that extended unsupervised food denial can be highly dangerous in the hands of the inexperienced. I am a well-known opponent of calorie reduction and the much-peddled obsession with how many calories a food contains. Persistent on/off low-calorie dieting is much abused but has never been a long-term answer to good health or sensible weight loss. However, I can find no evidence of either colonic irrigation or the type of gentle detox described here causing eating disorders.

- Colonic treatment could exacerbate existing inflammation.

  Qualified therapists take a detailed health history to enable them to decide whether or not a course of treatment is advisable. It is vital to give the practitioner as much information as possible about any surgical procedures, medical treatments, illnesses and current medication. Anyone with known or suspected bowel disease should approach pressurized colonic treatment with caution.

- Washing the bowel removes all the friendly flora so vital to good health.

  The treatment removes both good and bad bacteria. Replacement of the good bacteria, either using an anal implant or probiotic drink, is provided at each treatment. I would suggest asking for both the implant and the drink. Author's note: The protest about damage to beneficial bacteria seems quickly forgotten when the same objectors are issuing prescriptions for antibiotics!

- A high-fibre diet provides the same effect as colonic irrigation and is cheaper than specialist fibre products.

  My experience with patients has been that those who rely on wheat bran cereals as their main source of fibre do little to improve the internal health of the colon, often aggravating, rather than relieving, conditions such as IBS and diverticulitis. The results of increasing the intake of wheat bran can be bloating, flatulence, abdominal pain and intermittent diarrhoea and constipation. Wheat is an insoluble fibre which acts as a bulking agent but has no nutritional value. It helps to move recently collected wastes but does little or nothing to loosen old faeces. The exclusive use of insoluble (as opposed to soluble) fibre is now being questioned by some medical researchers. Greater improvements seem to be achieved using other forms of more gentle fibre in conjunction with dietary changes such as those recommended above and those used in the *Food Combining 2-Day Detox*.

Try the food-combining formula first. If you think you may need colonic treatment, contact The Colonic International Association, 31 Eton Hall, Eton College Road, London NW3 2DE. Telephone: 0171 483 1595. They will advise you of your nearest qualified practitioner.

Start Low – Go Slow

๑

The best of healers is good cheer
Proverb attributed to the Greek poet Pindar (518–438 BC)

Be gentle with yourself, and go slowly into your first detox session. Begin by spending the next two weeks cutting down on these items:

Alcohol	Fizzy drinks
Artificial sweeteners	Margarine-type spreads
Beef and pork products	Salt
Coffee	Sugar
Cola	Sugary foods
Cow's milk	Tea

Wheat-based products such as pastry and cake
Yeasty foods (including bread)

What's Left? Loads!

Promise yourself that, during these two weeks, you'll make a real effort to eat more healthily. Introduce extra fresh vegetables and salads, home-made vegetable soups, jacket potatoes (as long as they're organic), brown rice, live yoghurt, fresh oily fish, organic poultry and fresh fruit.

- Be really vigilant about washing fruits and vegetables before use.
- Choose organic produce whenever possible.
- Avoid any foods which you don't like or which you suspect may cause adverse reactions.
- Don't worry about food combinations at this point. We'll be introducing those later on.

DON'T FORGET THE WATER. No one will stay healthy for very long without water. Humans can live for weeks without food but will begin to suffer severe dehydration after only a matter of a day or two without water. During detox days, extra fluid is especially important to encourage toxins out of the system.

I really would very strongly recommend anyone to invest in a water filter. No need to opt for complicated under-sink units which cost a bomb and take up loads of cupboard space – a good quality jug or portable unit will perform quite well enough. Fill your kettle from your filter jug and use freshly filtered water for cooking and drinking. In fact, for everything except washing yourself, washing clothes and washing up! You'll find good-quality filter jugs in most supermarkets, hardware stores, kitchen shops and health stores.

One very important rule: remember to change the filter cartridge frequently and wash the jug thoroughly between each change. During use, keep the jug topped up so that water is always available. Neglected jugs and old cartridges will breed bacteria very quickly and the cartridge may not be effective if it is allowed to dry out.

If filtered water is not available, then choose non-carbonated bottled water. Unfiltered tap water is not recommended.

Two-day Detox Menu Planner

~

Effective health care depends upon self-care.
Ivan Illich from his book Medical Nemesis

For best results, to improve body function, speed elimination of wastes and boost energy levels, introduce two detox days into your regular routine every two to four weeks if you can – less often is still better than not at all. Ring the changes and vary the menus by referring to the alternative suggestions on pages 98–99. When you are comfortable with regular detoxification, you may decide to go for a slightly more stringent programme, in which case you can add Day Three.

Alternatively, use any of the days, singly or together, as a 'refresher' any time you are feeling sluggish, stressed, exhausted, need to recharge your batteries, or are suffering the effects of too many late nights or, indeed, any kind of excess. Read the whole of this section right through before you begin and make a shopping list of the items you are going to include for your first detox session. To maintain progress, follow the simple food-combining guidelines given from page 55. If you haven't food-combined before, it could be helpful, now, to turn to page 55 and remind yourself of those foods that combine well and those that do not. You'll also find food-combining guidelines alongside the main meal recipes below.

By all means use the programme on work days if that suits you. However, it's much better if you can find forty-eight hours when you're at home and under less pressure. At a weekend or during the week – it doesn't matter just as long as you give yourself priority. If you're really busy and feel that you can't fit the two days into your schedule, then follow the programme for one day this week and one day next week. This isn't quite as good but will still provide body benefits.

IMPORTANT: Ignore your usual set meal breaks during the detox. If you feel hungry any time between the recommended meals, then it's absolutely fine to tuck into any fresh fruit, vegetable or fruit juice, soup or herbal tea. It's important that you don't allow yourself to feel gnawingly empty.

For summer detox, I keep bottles of organic vegetable juice handy; health stores stock them. They provide tasty, nutritious and satisfying drinks. In the winter, warming and sustaining home-made vegetable soup makes a terrific pitstop.

What About Exercise?

Anyone who hasn't heard that regular exercise is good for their health must have just moved here from another planet. I don't need to tell you that walking, swimming, cycling and aerobics are all beneficial to the heart and circulation. Exercise also helps to detoxify the body and reduce acidity in the tissues. Rebounding (exercising on a mini-trampoline) is an excellent way to encourage lymph drainage and so is an added bonus to detoxification.

However, too much activity can be as dangerous as too little. Over-exercising can put strain on all body systems, in particular the immunity. During any detox programme, it is wiser to take a little less exercise. Fresh air, sunlight, a short brisk walk every day (or gentle rebounding if the weather is inclement) and plenty of deep breathing are all highly recommended. But don't jog for miles around the park or work out until you drop. It simply isn't necessary.

Before Bedtime on these Two Days

Add Geranium and Juniper essential oils to a warm bath and soak for ten minutes. See the chapter on essential oils which begins on page 120.

A couple of exercises that you should find helpful are deep breathing and abdominal massage.

Breathing is Cleansing

Deep breathing has major benefits and should be a fundamental part of any fitness programme. It cleanses, alkalizes, calms an overactive mind, enhances efficient cell turnover, improves the transport of oxygen and nutrients throughout the bloodstream, reduces anxiety and strengthens the lungs. (Our bodies know this. Think about how we 'sigh' at times of stress. And we even talk about 'taking a deep breath' before embarking on a major venture. But *don't* fall into the bad habit of only making 'a sharp intake of breath' – this *generates* stress!) Deep breathing also improves circulation and is a useful exercise for warming you up if you're chilled.

Each night before you go to sleep, practise breathing more deeply.
Lying on your back, make sure that you are comfortable and that every part of your body is as relaxed as possible.
Exhale completely.
Then inhale slowly, filling the lungs and pushing out your abdomen.
Hold for a count of two.
Then exhale slowly, releasing any pent-up tensions and anxieties. Picture the stress falling away from your body.
Repeat for ten in-breaths and ten out-breaths.

Abdominal Massage

Next, pressing firmly with your fingers, massage your abdominal area for a few minutes. Lubricate the skin with a little olive oil. Begin at the lower right side, just inside the right hip bone, and work your way upwards towards the waist, then across and down the left side. You should hear some gurgling and may pass trapped wind. This is a good sign and to be encouraged.

If you find the massage action hard work on your hands, use a soft rubber ball and roll it firmly over your abdomen in the same clockwise direction about 20 times. Or find a willing partner to do the massage for you. Abdominal massage is extremely beneficial if you suffer from constipation, IBS or candidiasis and could be likened to taking your intestines for a jog!

DAILY HEALING JUICE

Once each day, during your detox session, make up this healing juice. It makes a tasty aperitif while you are preparing the evening meal or a refreshing drink between meals.

For best results, you will need:

2 organic carrots, well scrubbed
1 or 2 apples, peeled
a couple of dozen grapes of any colour
1 raw beetroot, peeled
A few sprigs of parsley
A few sprigs of watercress or baby spinach leaves

Make sure the ingredients are washed really well. Then chop them all up and push them through your juicer or blender. Drink the results immediately but slowly, holding each sip in your mouth for a few seconds before swallowing. This recipe makes a good energy-boosting drink any time, is a terrific liver cleanser and is also excellent if you suspect a cold is lurking. If you are recovering from an ulcer or suffer with acid reflux or heartburn, try to drink the healing juice twice daily every day between meals; in other words, not just when you are following this detox. If you can't obtain all the ingredients, at least include the carrots, apples and grapes.

Fruit Suggestions

Use both fresh and dried fruit. Buy dried fruit in small quantities and use quickly. Avoid sprayed or glazed fruits (check labels for additives before you buy).

Apples
Apricots, fresh and dried
   Hunza apricots (from
   health-food stores)
Bananas
Blackberries
Blackcurrants
Blueberries
Cherries
Dates
Durian
Fig
Grapefruit
Grapes

Guava
Kiwi fruit
Lychee
Mango
Melon
Nectarines
Papaya (paw-paw)
Peaches
Pears
Pineapple
Pomegranates
Raspberries
– and anything else you
   can think of.

Salad Suggestions

Any fresh culinary herbs
Any kind of dark-leaf lettuce
Avocado pear
Baby spinach
Bell peppers (capsicums)
Black olives

Broccoli florets
Cauliflower florets
Celery
Chicory
Chinese leaves
Cucumber (without skin)

Vegetable Suggestions

Buy organic wherever you can, of course.

Any kind of beans	Ginger
Asparagus	Globe artichokes
Bamboo shoots	Jerusalem artichokes
Broccoli/calabrese	Leeks
Brussels sprouts	Marrow
Cabbage	Onions
Carrots	Potatoes
Cauliflower	Pumpkin (squash)
Cauliflower greens	Shallots
Celeriac	Spinach
Celery	Swede
Courgette (zucchini)	Turnip greens
Culinary herbs	Turnips
Garlic	

If you need oil for cooking, use extra-virgin olive oil.

Fenugreek seeds	Grated white cabbage
Grated carrot	Pumpkin seeds
Grated courgette	Rocket
Grated raw beetroot	Spanish (mild) onion
(avoid packaged pre-	Watercress
cooked beetroot)	Young dandelion greens

For dressings, use extra-virgin olive oil or cold-pressed safflower oil with organic cider vinegar, balsamic vinegar, fresh lemon juice or Bioforce Molkosan.

SPIRULINA FLAKES: For extra nourishment, sprinkle salads and soups with Spirulina flakes. In its organic form, this blue-green algae is a feast of nourishing nutrients including minerals and antioxidants. It contains high levels of beta-carotene and is one of the few vegetarian sources of Vitamin B12. Spirulina powder is useful for stirring into juice, and spirulina tablets are also available. Find it in your health store or check page 139 for stockist information.

Day One

First Thing in the Morning

Choose from these two drinks.

LEMON AND HONEY REFRESHER

To make this drink you will need:
The juice of 1 fresh lemon (organic if possible; remember
that pre-packed lemon juice contains preservative)
2 teaspoons of cold-pressed raw honey – preferably New
Zealand Manuka or similar (with honey there's a clear
relationship between cost and quality – the more
expensive the honey, the better it is)
250ml (approx. ¼pint) just boiled filtered water

Squeeze the lemon juice into a tumbler or large mug, add
the honey and pour on the boiled water. Stir until the
honey has dissolved.

GLASS OF DILUTED MOLKOSAN

Stir one tablespoon of Molkosan liquid (see note below)
into a glass of filtered or bottled water.

Whichever you choose, remember to sip slowly – don't
gulp. If you are short on time, take the drink with you
while you wash and dress.

MOLKOSAN is a Swiss drink made from whey, a by-product of cheese production. Don't worry, it doesn't taste cheesy! In fact, it has a very pleasant, slightly vinegary flavour. Molkosan makes a useful alternative to vinegar or lemon juice when making salad dressings and adds a piquancy to stir-fries and vegetable dishes. Medicines using whey have been popular for centuries and are said to have been favoured by the famous physicians of Ancient Greece, Hippocrates and Galen.

Internally, Molkosan is believed to have several benefits. It improves digestion, stimulates the immune system, regulates the metabolism and encourages a better balance of friendly flora in the gut. The drink also supplies a number of easily assimilated minerals. Dr Alfred Vogel – and Dr Verheyen whom I met on a fact-finding visit to Switzerland – both recommend the use of whey drinks for general health but particularly during any cleansing programme. Molkosan helps to alkalize the tissues, reducing acidity, and also improves bowel function. Overall, regular use of Molkosan seems to enhance energy levels.

Dosage: Mix one tablespoon of Molkosan with a tumbler of filtered or non-carbonated mineral water. Sip slowly before meals.

Molkosan is available from health stores. In case of difficulty, contact Bioforce at the address on page 141.

Day One Breakfast

FRESH FRUIT

Choose two or three pieces of your favourite fruit, washed and peeled, from the list on page 98. Eat as much as leaves you *comfortably* full. Help to cut the quantity of pesticide residues by peeling any fruit that isn't organic.

ORANGES and orange juice are best avoided. They are not included in the detox as they can cause headaches and digestive discomfort in some people.

Day One Mid-morning

ORGANIC LINSEEDS

Take 2 heaped teaspoons of organic linseeds with a
tumbler (large glass) of filtered water.
(See important notes below.)

LINSEEDS provide the body with soluble and insoluble fibre and vitamin-like substances called essential fatty acids. These are very easily damaged by exposure to heat, light and air. To ensure the best quality, choose only organic linseeds that are sold in sealed tubs or bags (such as Linoforce or Linusit Gold). Reseal the bag carefully after each opening or pour the contents into an airtight storage jar. Keep it in the refrigerator.

The fibre in linseeds is very gentle and easily dealt with by the body. Two daily heaped teaspoons with a large tumbler of water will coax a sluggish or irritable bowel to life and help remove wastes and poisons from the system. In very stubborn cases, it is perfectly acceptable to take two dessertspoons daily. Do remember, however, that to work properly and safely, fibre needs fluid. Don't take linseeds if you are not prepared to drink that tumbler of water. Check page 139's Directory for stockists of Linoforce or Linusit Gold.

Day One Lunch

SPINACH OMELETTE

This recipe follows food-combining guidelines by using egg (a first-class protein) with salad. There is no starch (bread, potatoes, rice or pasta) included with this meal.

You will need:
1 organic onion, peeled
2 large free-range eggs
(if possible find a local supplier who uses organic feed)
1 tablespoon of filtered water
Sea salt and freshly ground black pepper
Three good handfuls of baby spinach
(equivalent to one pre-packed bag)
1 tablespoon of extra-virgin olive oil

To prepare:

Chop the onion very finely.

Beat the eggs with the water, a little sea salt and black pepper.

Steam the spinach until just cooked (take care not to overcook). Put to one side.

Heat the olive oil in a frying pan and sauté the chopped onion until it softens. Pour in the egg mixture and cook until the omelette is set on the underside.

Spread the spinach over the upper surface and fold the omelette in half. Cover the pan and continue to cook the omelette for 1 further minute or until the egg is completely set.

Serve with a large freshly made salad. (Choose as many salad items as you like from the list on pages 98–99.)

Day One Mid-afternoon

A glass of filtered or bottled water or a cup of herb or fruit tea followed by

Half a dozen dried figs and a handful of unblanched almonds. Sweet, nourishing and filling.

TIP: Try to avoid very cold food and chilled drinks. They can disturb the digestion and liver function.

Day One Before Supper

If you haven't had your Healing Juice (see page 97) today, now would be a good time. Otherwise, enjoy a glass of vegetable or fruit juice or diluted Molkosan while you are preparing the meal.

Day One Supper

COLOURFUL RICE

This recipe follows food-combining guidelines by mixing the rice (a complex starch) with vegetables. There is no concentrated protein (ie meat, eggs or fish) served at this meal.

You will need:
2 tablespoons of extra-virgin olive oil
1 organic onion, peeled
1 clove fresh garlic, peeled and crushed
About ½ teaspoon of freshly grated ginger
1 good portion of cooked brown rice
1 organic carrot, scrubbed and finely grated
2 small organic tomatoes, chopped
½ small pepper (bell pepper or capsicum) – any colour,
cored, de-seeded and finely grated
2 tablespoons of frozen peas
1 tablespoon of sunflower seeds and/or pumpkin seeds
(mixed or separate)

To prepare:

In a wok or large pan suitable for stir-frying, heat the olive oil then saute the onion, crushed garlic and ginger until the onion is just tender.

Add the cooked rice, grated carrot, chopped tomatoes, grated pepper, peas and seeds. Keep the mixture moving over a hot ring for 5 minutes.

Serve with any kind of salad from your list on pages 98–99. Any leftovers can be served cold with salad tomorrow if you wish.

BROWN RICE is a great detoxifier and an excellent source of dietary fibre. It's also a very useful food for settling a sore stomach or calming an irritated digestive system. Also worth remembering is the fact that freshly cooked brown rice in its bland, plain and unflavoured state can be sustaining and soothing following a bout of nausea or food poisoning. However, cooked rice does not keep well. Always store leftovers in the coldest part of the refrigerator and use up within 24 hours.

Day One Before Bed

One or two bananas, mashed into a dish and drizzled with a little cold-pressed raw honey.

Day Two

First Thing in the Morning

Have the Lemon and Honey Refresher or the Molkosan on page 102.

Day Two Breakfast

FRESH FRUIT YOGHURT

You will need:
1 large carton (around 200g/7 oz) of plain sheep's or goat's yoghurt
1 ripe kiwi fruit, washed, sliced and peeled
1 apple, washed, sliced and peeled
1 teaspoon of cold-pressed raw honey
1 tablespoon of Spirulina flakes or powder

To prepare:
Put all the ingredients into a blender and mix into a smooth liquid. Drink at once.

Day Two Mid-morning

2 heaped teaspoons of linseeds with a tumbler of filtered water, as yesterday.

Day Two Lunch

SUMPTUOUS SALAD

Choosing ingredients from the Salad Suggestions on pages 98–99, create a sumptuous salad sprinkled with pine nuts and pumpkin seeds. For a tasty dressing, add a tablespoon of balsamic vinegar or Molkosan to a tablespoon of extra-virgin olive oil. Mix with a touch of dry mustard and black pepper and pour over the salad.

Day Two Mid-Afternoon

Two apples, washed well, peeled and sliced, along with Cup of herb or fruit tea, if desired.

Day Two Before Supper

Healing Juice (see page 97).

Day Two Supper

HALF AVOCADO PEAR FILLED WITH HUMMUS
followed by
JACKET POTATO

This supper follows food-combining guidelines by serving a starch (the potato) with vegetables or salad. There is no concentrated protein at this meal. Avocado pear combines well with either proteins or starches.

Have the avocado pear with hummus as your starter.

Then drizzle the baked jacket potato with extra-virgin olive oil and cider vinegar and eat it with salad or cooked vegetables. (Don't eat the potato skin unless it's organic.) If you have an oven timer, why not prepare the potato in the morning and set the cooker to switch on automatically? That way, supper is ready when you need it.

If you are pushed for time, have any Colourful Rice left over from yesterday, served with a big green salad.

Day Two Before Bed

Any fresh fruit.

AVOCADO If, at any time, you don't feel like eating a cooked meal, why not have a *whole* avocado with salad instead? Many people worry that avocados are fattening. They're not. They are simply full of nourishment, including monounsaturated oils, shown to be helpful to blood glucose levels *and* cholesterol balance.

Day Three

Only add day three if you feel you would like to extend your detox programme a little further.

First Thing in the Morning

Cup or glass of filtered water with a squeeze of fresh lemon juice *or* Kombucha Tea.

KOMBUCHA is a fermented tea that contains a range of vitamins, minerals, amino acids and enzymes. Kombucha itself is a fungus. Sounds strange? Well, it's been used for centuries as a healing, revitalizing drink. Particularly well known across Asia, its first use can be traced back to around 200 BC. Now available in the West as a health supplement, research demonstrates that it can enhance athletic performance and has helped those suffering from a variety of health problems, including fatigue and digestive difficulties. It is also said to be a terrific detoxifier. I find it a refreshing alternative to other beverages. It has a very pleasant flavour, not unlike cider. If you like the taste, take a 150ml measure of Kombucha (half of one small bottle) first thing in the morning and another 150ml last thing at night. Don't forget to sip the drink slowly.

Kombucha is available from health stores. In case of difficulty, page 139 has stockist information.

Day Three Breakfast

Any kind of fresh fruit in any quantity. (Choose from the list on page 98.)
Cup of Bambu or herbal tea.

BAMBU is a coffee substitute prepared from organically grown chicory, figs, malted barley, gluten-free wheat and acorns. It contains no caffeine and no artificial chemicals or preservatives. Because it is gluten-free and organic, the wheat in Bambu does not appear to cause the adverse reactions associated with bread wheat. Try a small amount of Bambu (say, half a teaspoonful) before making a full-size cup. Some health stores stock one-cup sachets. Best taken black.

Day Three Mid-morning

2–3 heaped teaspoons of organic linseeds with a large tumbler of water.

Day Three Lunch

Glass of diluted Molkosan or Kombucha Tea, followed by Large portion of salad made from any of the ingredients in your salad list (pages 98–99). Serve with a chunk of goat's cheese (available from supermarkets, health stores and delicatessens).

GOAT'S CHEESE is a major protein food and digests well if combined with salad but does not mix comfortably with starchy foods.

Day Three Mid-afternoon

Glass of Molkosan or herbal tea.

Day Three Before Supper

Healing Juice (see page 97).

Day Three Supper

HOME-MADE VEGETABLE SOUP

This recipe includes potato, which means that this is a starch-based meal.

You will need:
1 tablespoon of extra-virgin olive oil
1 organic onion, peeled and chopped
1 clove garlic, peeled and crushed
1 head of broccoli
2 organic carrots
1 turnip
1 organic potato
1 pinch of freshly grated nutmeg
Filtered water

To Prepare:

Heat the olive oil in a large saucepan and fry the chopped onion and crushed garlic for a couple of minutes.

Wash and chop the vegetables into small pieces and add to the pan with the nutmeg. Keep them moving over the heat for 5 minutes.

Then add enough water to cover and simmer until the carrot is tender.

Allow to cool until safe enough to liquidize. Blend to the preferred consistency – chunky or smooth. Reheat and serve at once.

VEGETABLE SOUP: Freshly prepared home-made vegetable soup is a superstore of vitamins, minerals, dietary fibre and valuable fluid. Do try to make your own whenever you can. The recipe given here is very simple and not a bit time-consuming. If you truly don't have time to make your own soup, then choose one of the fresh vegetable soups that are now available in cartons. Make sure that you buy additive-free brands that contain only the freshest ingredients, such as those produced by the New Covent Garden Soup Company (or supermarket own brand equivalent). Dried or canned soups are *not* suitable and should be avoided. They are likely to contain high levels of either sugar or salt and may also include anti-caking agents and a range of other additives. In addition, the canning and drying processes destroy significant amounts of nourishment.

Other Lunch and Supper Suggestions

To vary your two- or three-day programme, you can substitute any of these dishes at lunch or supper time:

Grated apple and grated carrot with chopped celery and walnuts, dressed with extra-virgin olive oil and lemon juice.

Pumpkin seeds with any finely shredded dark green lettuce, watercress, rocket, grated cabbage and chopped cucumber (without skin).

Avocado pear served with hummus. Use half or a whole avocado, depending upon the size of your appetite. Simply fill the hollow(s) in the cut avocado with hummus and then tuck in. If you have half left-over, wipe the cut surface with lemon juice, wrap well and refrigerate. It will keep until the next day.

Sliced avocado and skinned tomato with chopped bell peppers and any chopped fresh herbs.

Apple chunks with dried figs and nuts. Slice and peel two apples. Serve with half a dozen dried figs and a handful of walnut or pecan halves.

Big tomato salad. Skinned, sliced tomatoes with chopped basil, parsley and cold-pressed safflower oil. This is also great with chopped mint and balsamic vinegar.

Grated apple, raw beetroot, carrot and watercress.

Sticks of carrot and celery, fresh radish and broccoli or cauliflower florets dipped in curd cheese or hummus.

Any vegetable stir-fry (cook with extra-virgin olive oil).

A medley of steamed or gently boiled vegetables sprinkled with lemon juice and a little sea salt.

A large bowl of home-made vegetable soup.

A large bowl of sheep's or goat's yoghurt mixed with a little cold-pressed raw honey, flaked almonds or fresh fruit.

> Food-combining guidelines: yoghurt is a protein food. Some food-combining experts do not recommend that proteins are taken with fruit because proteins take much longer to digest than fruit; a combination which could cause fermentation and indigestion in some people. However, sheep's and goat's yoghurt are unusual in that they are quick and easy to digest, combining happily with fruit. If you choose yoghurt as a dessert, remember that it's fine after a protein meal but isn't such a good idea after a starch meal.

Going Out

You don't have to stay at home to eat healthily. The following pages give you tips for when travelling and eating out.

Food Tips For Travelling and Eating Out

꒛

If you are away from home a great deal and forced to rely on food which is prepared for you by others – or if your job means you must eat out regularly – you can still make moves towards a healthier eating programme. For example:

- Always carry fresh water and snacks with you in the car. Mix up a bag of sunflower seeds, pumpkin seeds, almonds and dried fruit. Or buy a pack of cereal bars from the health-food shop. If you know you are going on a long car trip, prepare a salad in a cold carrier or soup in an insulated flask to take with you.
- Whilst waiting for restaurant, hotel or café meals to be served, ask for a large tumbler of mineral water (preferably *not* fizzy) and drink this before the meal.
- Choose fruit or vegetable soup as a light entrée.
- Say no to the bread roll.
- Refuse the fries.
- Some restaurants seem to serve plenty of potato but use other root or green vegetables – or salad – only as garnish. (If your meal contains protein, skip the

spuds.) Ask what vegetables will accompany the meal and order extra portions.

- For even more fresh nourishment, request a good-sized side salad with olive oil and vinegar or lemon juice dressing.
- Say no to mayonnaise.
- Go for grilled fish, poultry or seafood dishes – or lean lamb.
- Ring the changes by asking for the vegetarian options.
- To cut down the risk of overeating (and reduce the cost), why not choose two entrées instead of an entrée and a main course. Or ask for children's portions.
- Pass on the rich sauces and sugary desserts.
- Leave a little time between courses.
- Most hotels are happy to make up packed lunches if you warn them the night before. Healthy options are nearly always available. Where they aren't, try to extend their imagination beyond cheese and ham sandwiches and white bread by asking for fresh fruit, dried fruit, nuts, seeds, crudités, salad, seafood, cold chicken, yoghurt and bottled water. Could they fill your flask with hot soup? If you are returning to the same place that night, they may lend you a flask if you don't have your own.
- Remember that, while you are what you eat, you are *where* you eat, too. If a hostelry or restaurant seems reluctant to provide healthy choices or to accommodate special needs, go somewhere else. I remember staying at one very grand watering hole where a request for the vegetarian option was met with a blank stare followed

by much head shaking, a ten-minute summit meeting between chef and waiter and the grudging offer of a cheese omelette! Needless to say, I didn't go there again.

The Benefits of Pure Essential Oils

❧

How beautiful it is to do nothing and then rest afterward.

Spanish proverb

Throughout the *Food Combining 2-Day Detox*, we've talked a lot about the benefits of healthy eating and how changing the diet can reduce toxic overload. We've also looked at how other factors in a frantic lifestyle can be amended to reduce stress and help our exhausted bodies to work more efficiently. One area that contributes hugely to long-term protection is the use of essential oils, familiar to most of us through aromatherapy. Most people know the names of at least one or two essential oils and, perhaps, their uses. Until I began to try out different oils and read more about them, I had no idea that they had so many healing talents. These are just a few:

Antibacterial
Antidepressant
Antifungal
Anti-inflammatory
Antiseptic
Antispasmodic

Antiviral

Astringent

Balancing

Calming

Comforting

Confidence boosting

Decongesting

Deodorizing

De-stressing

Diuretic

Immune-boosting

Invigorating

Pain-relieving

Relaxing

Sedating

Sensual

Skin-conditioning

Sleep-inducing

Soothing

Stimulating

Uplifting

CLEANSING
and
DETOXIFYING

So where do they come from?

The concentrated essential oils used in aromatherapy are extracted from the seeds, flowers, fruit, leaves, peel, roots, grasses and woods of a wide variety of aromatic plants. Each oil has its own unique *aroma* and healing properties and may contain a hundred or more different chemical constituents. Some oils are recommended for use only by a qualified therapist but others are eminently suitable for home use.

History

The use of fragrant plant extracts dates back several thousand years. In ancient Egypt, for example, Cedar oil was used for religious ceremonies and in perfume, and Frankincense was favoured as a calming, clearing essence.

However, it is only over the last hundred years that experts have learned about the chemistry behind the extraordinary properties of these plant extracts.

It is said to be the French researcher René Gattefosse who coined the now familiar word *Aromatherapy*. The story goes that in the 1930s, when he was working in the laboratory of a perfume company, he sustained a severe burn on his hand. Almost without thinking, he plunged it into the nearest bowl of liquid – which just happened to be essential oil of Lavender. The damage healed with exceptional speed and almost no scarring. His experience led him to study in depth the properties of other oils. Another Frenchman, Dr Jean Valnet, discovered the healing power of essential oils while working as a surgeon during the Second World War, when other medicines were in short supply. Since then, a number of eminent researchers have continued to investigate and validate these valuable essences.

The Importance of Odour

The human sense of smell is acute. Odours and aromas evoke memories and emotions and can influence a person's mood, attitude and even efficiency. The use of the right blend of essential oils in the workplace is known to boost productivity and improve concentration. Research also shows that essential oils have the power to influence all body systems including the nervous system and immunity. When used particularly in conjunction with massage, the right choice of oils encourages effective lymph drainage and other important eliminative processes.

How to use Essential Oils

In Massage

One of the best ways to familiarize yourself with essential oils is to use them for home massage. The simplest method is to mix two drops of your chosen oil with 5ml (one teaspoon) of carrier oil (see the box on page 126). Warm the oil in the hands before applying to the body.

Don't massage if there is fever or high temperature, varicose veins, skin inflammation, broken skin or recent fractures.

For Bathing

Add a few drops of diluted oil to the bath before you get in. On detox days, use oils that cleanse, purify and balance such as Juniper, Geranium and Clary Sage. Before bed, choose relaxing oils like Lavender and Chamomile. In the morning, revive with refreshing, invigorating oils: for example, Tangerine, Pine or Rosemary. To energize, try Rosemary with Lemon.

For A Relaxing Footbath

Add three drops of Lavender and three drops of Lemon Grass to a bowl of warm water deep enough to immerse the feet and ankles. Sit and read, watch TV or just rest until the water begins to cool. Then dry the feet with a warm towel. If feet are tired and you are exhausted but you have to find the energy from somewhere to go out in the evening, a footbath using Lavender with three drops of Peppermint can relieve aches and pains and stimulate the system.

Fill the Air with Fragrance

Add a few drops of oil to a burner or aromastream. The simplest (and least expensive) method of vaporizing is to choose a burner. These are usually made of pottery with a lower compartment for a nightlight or small candle and an upper section (or detachable saucer) to hold the water and the oil. The heat of the candle slowly evaporates the water and releases the aroma of the essential oil into the atmosphere. There are some very attractive and colourful styles available but, when buying, do consider practicalities as well as aesthetics. Choose a design that has a deep 'well' as these hold more water and do not dry out. Shallow burners tend to vaporise all their water before the candle gives out, increasing the risk of the burner cracking. For the nearest stockists of quality products, contact the companies listed on page 139.

Here are a few suggestions on which oils to choose:

- On detox days, burn Clary Sage, Juniper, Geranium and Tangerine. Or Pine and Eucalyptus.
- If you are suffering with a cold, catarrh or fuzzy head, try Eucalyptus with Lemon Grass or Eucalyptus with Lemon.
- If your confidence needs boosting, use Sandalwood and Rosemary.
- To stir the thought processes into gear first thing in the morning, choose Peppermint with Lavender or Rosemary with Juniper. If my concentration is flagging, I find that Orange and Grapefruit oils are a good combination.
- Peppermint on its own can clear a headache.
- On a chilly day, mix Orange with Ginger.
- To relax and unwind in the evening, burn Frankincense with Rosewood.

Add to Paper Tissues or Hankies

Add a drop or two of oil to a handkerchief or tissue amd place it in your pocket or under the pillow at night. Lavender and Frankincense are relaxing after a stressful day. Eucalyptus helps if you are confined to bed with a cold. Ylang-Ylang is the oil for passion!

CARRIER OILS

Carrier or base oils are those used to dilute the essential oils for massage purposes. Always choose the best quality cold-pressed oils. Carrier oils should also be of the highest quality, purchased in dark glass bottles and stored with similar care. Their shelf life may be limited – between six months and one year. Never buy oils of any kind in clear or plastic containers.

Use **Avocado Oil** if you are treating dry skin or arthritic conditions.

Evening Primrose Oil can be a valuable base oil when treating hormonal imbalances or skin problems such as eczema and psoriasis.

Extra-Virgin Olive Oil is the best choice for abdominal massage or as a 'hot-oil hair conditioner'. To condition the hair, place 1 tablespoon of olive oil in an egg cup in a bowl of hot water. When the oil is heated through, rub it into the hair, wrap a towel around, and relax for 10 minutes or so. Shampoo out.

Grapeseed Oil is a good oil for general use, light and easily absorbed.

Sweet Almond Oil, extracted from the almond kernel, is also light and easily absorbed. It contains several valuable nutrients including vitamins A, B1, B6 and E.

Wheatgerm Oil is the best choice for healing scar tissue as it is rich in Vitamin E. However, it may not be suitable for anyone with a sensitivity or allergy to wheat.

Try **Apricot Kernel Oil** if the skin is inflamed or very sensitive. It's also very kind to older skins.

Combinations

Every expert I've ever talked to about essential oils seems to have varying views on which oils mix best with each other. Choice depends to a very great extent on personal preference. The prevailing circumstances or condition being treated are also taken into account. The list below is a guide only and, because of limitations of space, cannot include all the oils that are available. When I began to learn about and use essential oils at home, I started with half a dozen different oils and found out as much as possible about each one before investing in further purchases. You might like to do the same. It is a fascinating subject.

Try	With
Cedarwood	Eucalyptus, Geranium or Sandalwood
Chamomile	Geranium, Lavender or Ylang-Ylang
Clary Sage	Rosemary or Ylang-Ylang
Cypress	Frankincense, Juniper or Lemon
Eucalyptus	Cedarwood, Marjoram or Rosemary
Frankincense	Cypress, Orange, Lavender, Ginger or Grapefruit
Geranium	Cypress, Lavender, Juniper or Rosemary
Ginger	Frankincense, Marjoram or Orange
Grapefruit	Frankincense
Juniper	Frankincense, Lavender, Lemon or Lemon Grass
Lavender	mixes with most oils and is especially good in relaxing blends
Lemon	Chamomile, Frankincense, Juniper or Lavender
Lemon Grass	Eucalyptus
Mandarin	Rosewood or Ylang-Ylang
Marjoram	Ginger
Orange	Frankincense, Ginger, Patchouli or Ylang-Ylang
Peppermint	Rosemary or Ginger
Rosemary	Cedarwood, Frankincense, Geranium or Juniper
Rosewood	Mandarin or Ylang-Ylang

Sandalwood	Cypress, Lavender or Cedarwood
Tea Tree	Use alone or with Pine or Eucalyptus
Ylang-Ylang	Clary Sage, Lavender, Lemon or Patchouli

My grateful thanks to Nelson & Russell, Natural by Nature Oils and Jurlique for their suggestions and advice.

Caring for your Oils

Proper storage is vital if the beneficial properties of the oil are to be maintained. Once opened, the oil lasts around eighteen months. Unopened, the contents should remain effective for up to three years. Citrus oils, like Lemon, Grapefruit and Orange, are the least stable and have a shorter life of around six months. Quality oils will always be sold in dark glass bottles with good screw caps. Store the bottles in a cool, dark place and always replace the cap as soon as you have taken what you need. If exposed to light and air, the oils will be damaged and will evaporate to nothing. Don't keep your oils near to homoeopathic medications.

Buy small quantities of individual oils or blends and replace them as necessary. Somewhere on the label should be the words 'Pure Essential Oil'. The term 'Aromatherapy Oil' on its own does not necessarily mean that the oils are pure; they may have a pleasant smell but provide little or nothing in the way of therapeutic properties. There are some reports of unpleasant skin reactions being caused by impure oils.

Pure quality essential oils are likely to vary in price between one essence and another, cost being determined by the scarcity of the plant and the time involved in distillation. Ranges of oils that are all similarly priced are unlikely to be pure.

Good brands to look out for are:

Jurlique (from the Naturopathic Health and Beauty Company on 0181 995 3948)

Natural by Nature Oils (0181 202 5718)

Gerard House (from English Grains on 01283 228344)

Nelson & Russell (0181 780 4200 for trade enquiries or 0171 495 2404 for general enquiries)

Tisserand (01273 206640)

TWELVE TOP OILS

The twelve oils described below formed the basis of my original 'collection' and are my first choice for any first-aid cabinet. Frankincense, Orange and Ylang-Ylang are my absolute favourites simply because they smell sensational. I wouldn't be without Juniper, Geranium or Clary Sage, especially on detox days. Eucalyptus improves breathing and clears a stuffy head. Ginger is invaluable in chilly weather, for warming a cold body. Lavender oil is an essential in the kitchen for minor scalds and burns, but is also great if I can't get to sleep. Marjoram is one of the best for aches and pains. Peppermint is for headaches and aching feet. Tea Tree is an amazing antiseptic.

Clary Sage (*Salvia sclarea*) is a herb found in Mediterranean regions. Distilled from the whole plant, the aroma is warm and woody. This balancing, mood-lifting oil is valuable for anyone suffering from:

Muscle cramps

Negative thoughts

Physical exhaustion from overwork

Premenstrual tension

Restlessness or

Stress

Eucalyptus (*Eucalyptus globulus*) Native to Australia and one of the tallest trees in the world, the Eucalyptus essence is extracted mainly from its leaves. The deep and penetrating aroma is useful as an inhalation, chest rub and room freshener. Eucalyptus is famed for its strongly antiseptic and antiviral properties, and is effective for all kinds of infections and for breathing and respiratory problems, including:

Asthma

Bronchitis

Catarrh

Colds

Influenza and

Sinusitis

It's also valuable for easing the symptoms of Shingles, Chickenpox and Cold Sores.

Head lice hate Eucalyptus!

Frankincense (*Boswellia thurifera*) The soothing scent of Frankincense is probably my all-time favourite. Native to North and East Africa, the oil is distilled from the resin which exudes from its bark. Chosen traditionally for religious services, it is *the* oil to help someone cope with bereavement, and to calm fears and insecurities (especially at night). Blended with Grapefruit oil, I found it especially helpful for soothing the emotional distress, despondency and confusion that I felt when my first husband died. Frankincense also improves breathing, enhances concentration and has a 'protective' quality which eases the trauma of excessively stressful situations. A good skin oil, too; add one drop to your favourite night cream and massage into the face before bedtime. Use this oil if you are a 'shivery' type who feels the cold at night.

Geranium (*Pelargonium graveolens*) Geraniums are native to South Africa but are also very familiar herbaceous plants in this country. Geranium is balancing, regulating and uplifting but also useful as a sedative for anyone who is overanxious. Good for hormonal disorders such as PMTS, menopausal disturbance, difficult periods and for relieving fluid retention. Geranium is cleansing and balancing for both excessively dry and very oily skin. Add one or two drops to a carrier oil and use for gentle facial massage or shake a similar amount into skin tonic and wipe over the face with a cottonwool pad. Use Geranium on your detox days.

Ginger (*Zingiber officinale*) The essence of this deliciously warm oil comes from the rhizome. Apart from being well known as a treatment for nausea and digestive upsets, ginger is the most wonderful oil for winter use, especially if you come home feeling chilled to the marrow or soaked from the rain. Put a couple of drops in a warm bath and see how it eases the aches and pains of rheumatism, colds and flu. With Marjoram – and added to a carrier oil – it is extremely soothing when massaged into the abdomen to relieve tummy ache or period pains. Ginger is a strong oil and should only ever be used in the smallest quantities.

Juniper (*Juniperus communis*) This essential oil is distilled from its berries, the same berries as are used in gin making. The cleansing action of Juniper makes it a powerful diuretic, excellent kidney tonic and blood purifier, and useful for treating fluid retention and cystitis. *However, it is not suitable for use on anyone with kidney disease.* Juniper can help skin problems – including acne and eczema – as well as the aches and pains of arthritis and rheumatism. A good choice if you are feeling lethargic or vulnerable. Use Juniper on your detox days.

Lavender (*Lavendula officinalis*) Probably the most versatile of all the essential oils, Lavender has a wide range of therapeutic properties. Soothing for all kinds of emotional imbalance, it is sedating, neutralizing and harmonizing. Lavender stimulates the immune system, and can be used in wound healing, to reduce scarring, on boils and on insect bites. Its analgesic and cooling actions make it valuable for painful joints, headaches and burns – including sunburn. Considered a very safe oil, suitable for babies and young children, Lavender is one of the few that can be applied neat if necessary. Lavender mixes well with – and enhances the action of – most other oils.

Marjoram (*Origanum marjorana*) A common garden herb with a host of helpful talents, the oil is distilled from the whole plant which has a medicinal and camphorous aroma. An antispasmodic and so one of the best oils for treating muscular aches and pains. On the emotional side, marjoram is comforting and reduces nervousness, irritability and anxiety. Valuable to anyone with pre-menstrual problems, period pains or heavy monthly bleeding.

Orange (*Citrus sinensis*) Essential oil of orange is expressed from the peel. Not surprisingly, the essence is refreshing and stimulating, and also a mood enhancer. Orange oil is the best choice for burning in any room where there is to be a party or celebration. A good 'wake-up' oil for the bath but be sure to use it in low concentrations because too much might cause skin irritation.

Caution: Mix with a little water and patch test first. Not suitable for sensitive skins or for children.

Peppermint (*Mentha piperita*) The familiar fresh, minty aroma of peppermint oil comes from the whole plant. Used most commonly for treating digestive disorders, irritable bowel syndrome, headaches and sinus problems. Also a nerve tonic, peppermint is useful for calming anxiety *and* for lifting depression. Peppermint oil in a vaporizer clears a stuffy atmosphere and deters biting insects such as mosquitoes. In a footbath, it will refresh and sweeten tired, sticky feet.

Caution: this is a strong oil. Use it sparingly. Don't use it at the same time as homoeopathic medicines as it may counteract their effect.

Tea Tree (*Melaleuca alternifolia*) The essential oil of the tea tree is distilled from the leaves and produces a distinctive and very recognizable medicinal odour. Native to South Eastern Australia, the plant extracts have been used for centuries by the Australian Aborigines. Tea tree has exceptionally powerful antibacterial, antiviral and antifungal properties, and is one of the best treatments for thrush, fungal infections of the nails and for athlete's foot. Tea Tree oil has so many useful properties that it is, not surprisingly, being dubbed 'the first aid kit in a bottle', useful for cuts, grazes, bruises, sprains, burns, stings, spots and pimples, cold sores, verrucae and warts. It is an immune system stimulant and may be particular helpful in glandular fever. Thursday Plantation Tea Tree products are available from health stores, pharmacies and Boots.

Manuka is the Maori name given to New Zealand Tea Tree Oil. Manuka oil is also highly recommended and comes in strong and mild versions. Manex Manuka can be found in good independent health stores. In case of difficulty, contact New Zealand Natural Food Company on 0181 961 4410.

Ylang-Ylang (*Cananga odorata*) The name (pronounced 'Ill-ang Ill-ang') means Flower of Flowers. One of the most sensuous and exotic of perfumes, Ylang-Ylang oil is distilled from its beautiful yellow flowers. Best known for its balancing effect on heart rhythm and respiration, Ylang-Ylang is also sedating for the nervous system. Use it to calm and quieten, following severe trauma or shock, and to cool anger. Ylang-Ylang is confidence-boosting and effective at helping sexual difficulties such as frigidity and impotence. Use it with Patchouli (in a vaporizer and in the bathwater) if you are planning the night of your dreams! Use sparingly. Too much can cause a headache.

WANT TO KNOW MORE?

It's good to have a quick and easy reference to hand if you want to know which essential oil is best for any particular condition. For safety's sake, it makes sense to learn about any oil that you decide to try. If you don't wish to buy a whole range of different oils, choose ready-mixed blends instead. Page 000 has details.

Three of the best little books available are these:

1. *Aromatherapy For You At Home* by Franzesca Watson £2.99 including postage from Natural by Nature Oils, 9 Vivian Avenue, Hendon Central, London NW4 3UT.

2. *Aromatherapy: A Nurses Guide For Women* by Ann Percival (£2.99).
3. *Aromatherapy – A Guide For Home Use* by Christine Westwood (£1.99) which explains how to make up massage blends and beauty treatments. Available from health stores, bookshops and some chemists. Or by mail from the publisher on 01483 570821.

For more detailed information, including over 800 'recipes' for everyday use, *Aromatherapy Blends and Remedies* by Franzesca Watson (published by Thorsons £8.99) is highly recommended.

For Safety's Sake

Essential oils are strong and need to be treated with respect. The following precautions should be noted:

Always follow the pack instructions on recommended quantities.

Don't be tempted to use more than is recommended. Twice the quantity will not produce twice the benefit.

Don't apply oils directly to the skin without first diluting them in a carrier oil.

Keep essential oils away from the eyes.

Never take oils internally!

Treat essential oils as you would medicines and keep containers well away from inquisitive children and pets!

If you are pregnant, seek professional advice from a qualified practitioner before using essential oils. Some are not suitable for use during pregnancy.

Detox Directory

๛

Special foods, supplements and equipment

For the following products, first of all try your local health store. In case of difficulty, contact the company by post or telephone: the addresses follow on page 140.

Bambu Coffee Alternative
Bleach-free sanitary protection
Boldocynara Tincture
Essential oils
Gluten-free foods
Herbal preparations including Silymarin (Milk Thistle)
Honey
Jurlique Body Contouring Gel (see Naturopathic Health & Beauty Company – page 144)
Kenwood water filters
Kombucha Tea
Linoforce
Linusit Gold Linseeds
Liver Herbs
Molkosan
Psyllium Husk Fibre Capsules
Regular 10 Fibre Supplement

Skin brushes
Spirulina flakes, tablets or powder
Wheat-free foods

The following companies supply, in addition to items
mentioned specifically in this book, a wide range of
vitamin, mineral and other health-related products:

Bioforce
Blackmores
FSC (Food Supplement Company)
Gerard House
Larkhall Green Farm
Natural by Nature
Natural Flow
Naturopathic Health & Beauty Company
Nelson & Russell
Pharma Nord
Solgar
Xynergy

Biocare (*Mail order only*)
    Biocare Ltd
    Lakeside
    180 Lifford Lane
    Kings Norton
    Birmingham B30 3NT
    Telephone: 0121 433 3727

Suppliers of:
Silymarin Complex (Milk Thistle)
Antioxidants
Colon Care Capsules
Garlicin garlic capsules
Vitamin C
Enzyme-Activated B Complex
Adult One-Daily Vitamins and Minerals (contains B vitamins)
Bio-acidophilus

Bioforce:
  Bioforce
  Olympic Business Park
  Dundonald
  Ayrshire KA2 9BE
  Telephone: 01563 851177

Suppliers of:
Boldocynara liver and gallbladder drops
Echinaforce
Linoforce
Bambu coffee
Organic seasonings
Molkosan lacto-fermented whey

Blackmores:
  House of Blackmores
  37 Rothschild Road

Chiswick
London W4 5HT
Telephone: 0181 987 8640

Suppliers of:
Garlix garlic tablets
Bio-C Low Acid formula Vitamin C Complex
Executive Formula B (also contains Vitamin C)
Acidophilus and Bifidus
Organic Spirulina Crystal Flakes and tablets

Bodywise:
Bodywise UK Ltd
14 Lower Court Road
Almondsbury
Bristol BS12 4DX
Telephone: 01454 615500

Suppliers of:
Bleach-free sanitary protection

FSC (Food Supplement Company):
FSC Information Centre
The Health & Diet Company
Europa Park
Stoneclough Road
Radcliffe
Manchester M26 1GG
Telephone: 01204 707420

Suppliers of:
Linusit Gold Linseeds
Herbal tinctures
Milk Thistle (Silymarin)
Vitamin C
Multivitamin/minerals
Antioxidants

Kenwood Water Filters:
  Kenwood Ltd
  New Lane
  Havant
  Hampshire
  PO9 2NH
  Telephone: 01705 476000

Kombucha Tea is available from:
  Natural Health Products
  11 Railway Street
  Lisburn
  County Antrim BT28 1XG
  Telephone: 01846 662551

Larkhall Green Farm:
  Larkhall Green Farm
  225 Putney Bridge Road
  London SW15 2PY
  Telephone: 0181 874 1130

Suppliers of:
Natural Flow Psyllium Husk Fibre Capsules
Skin brushes
Regular 10 Fibre Supplement with herbs and acidophilus

The Naturopathic Health & Beauty Company:
   Naturopathic Health & Beauty Company
   37 Rothschild Road
   Chiswick
   London W4 5HT
   Telephone: 0181 995 3948

Suppliers of:
Jurlique Body Contouring Gel
Jurlique Pure Essential Oils

New Zealand Natural Food Company:
   New Zealand Natural Food Company
   Unit 7, 55–57 Park Royal Road
   London NW10 7JP
   Telephone 0181 961 4410

Suppliers of:
Cold-pressed raw organic honey

Pharma Nord UK:
   Pharma Nord UK Ltd
   Telford Court
   Morpeth
   Northumberland NE61 2DB
   Telephone 0800 591756 or 01670 519989

Suppliers of:
Antioxidants
Vitamin C

Solgar:
   Solgar Vitamins
   Aldbury
   Tring
   Hertfordshire HP23 5PT
   Telephone: 01442 890335

Suppliers of:
Multivitamins/minerals
Antioxidants
Vitamin C
Herbal preparations

Xynergy Health Products:
   Xynergy Health Products
   Ash House
   Stedham
   Midhurst
   West Sussex GU29 0PT
   Telephone: 01730 813642

Suppliers of:
   Spirulina powder and tablets

Food Allergies and Sensitivities

For those with food allergies and sensitivities and anyone who prefers to avoid gluten and wheat, the following addresses may be useful:

Berrydales Newsletter (*The Inside Story*) is published quarterly and is full of wonderful recipes and relevant health information. Send an s.a.e. for subscription details.
Berrydale Publishers
Berrydale House
5 Lawn Road
London NW3 2XS

For stockist details on a range of specialist food products, contact:
Kjaers Food For Life
The Old Chapel
Drury Lane
Mortimer
Berkshire RG7 2JN
Telephone and fax: 0118 933 1273
and
Virani Food Products
10–14 Stewarts Road
Finedone Road Industrial Estate
Wellingborough
Northamptonshire NN8 4RJ
Telephone: 01933 276483

For free-range and organic meat, poultry and vegetables, Contact:

The Soil Association
86 Colston Street
Bristol
Avon BS1 5BB
Telephone: 0117 929 0661

They will give details of stockists in your area. They also provide lists of farms and other outlets that sell approved organic produce. Some companies will deliver to your door.

Most major supermarkets stock some organic produce. If there is something they don't have that you need, then it really is worth asking. I have found Tesco and Waitrose both particularly helpful.

Tests available for nutritional deficiencies, food allergies:

BIOLAB
9 Weymouth Street
London W1N 3FF
Telephone: 0171 636 5905/5959

Tests also available to qualified practitioners via:

BIOCARE
Lakeside
180 Lifford Lane
Kings Norton
Birmingham B30 3NT
Telephone: 0121 433 3727

Inform Yourself

FLAG (The Food Labelling Agenda)
For further information, send a stamped addressed envelope to:
  The FLAG Administrator
  PO Box 105
  Hampton
  Middlesex TW12 3TL

COLONIC THERAPY:
For further information, contact:
  The Colonic International Association
  31 Eton Hall
  Eton College Road
  London NW3 2DE
  Telephone: 0171 483 1595

For information on medical treatments, drug side effects and alternative therapies, subscribe to these journals:
WHAT DOCTORS DON'T TELL YOU
and
PROOF!
Both available from:
  Wallace Press
  4 Wallace Road
  London N1 2PG
Send an s.a.e. for information.

Recommended Reading

ﾟ

The books and journals in this list are those that I have found indispensable, fascinating reading. They can be ordered either directly from bookshops or via the addresses given or from local libraries.

The Food Magazine. Quarterly journal packed with information about the food we eat and where it comes from. For details, send an s.a.e. to The Food Commission, 3rd Floor, Worship Street, London EC2A 2BH.

The Food We Eat by Joanna Blythman. An essential guide to healthier food choices and tips on how to recognize the good and the bad. An honest assessment of the way in which much of our food is produced and marketed. An absorbing book for anyone who really cares about what they buy in the supermarket and grocery store.
Published by Michael Joseph
ISBN 0 7181 39127

The Killing of the Countryside by Graham Harvey. A no-holds barred documentary of the scandal of farming subsidies and the damage caused by the chemical overload of our land.

Published by Jonathan Cape
ISBN 0 224 04444 3

Food and Healing by Annemarie Colbin. For anyone who wonders why, in this era of advanced medicine, we still suffer so much serious illness.
Published by Ballantine Books
ISBN 0 345 30385 7

Food Combining in 30 Days by Kathryn Marsden. The bestselling step-by-step guide to simple food combining and healthy weight control.
Published by Thorsons
ISBN 0 7225 2960 0

The Beauty Bible by Sarah Stacey and Josephine Fairley. The ultimate beauty handbook packed with tips on every aspect of skin care. Highly recommended.
Published by Kyle Cathie
ISBN Hardback 1 85626 255 1
ISBN Paperback 1 85626 267 7

Aromatherapy for You at Home by Franzesca Watson. A beginner's guide. Highly recommended.
Cost £2.99 including postage and packing from Natural by Nature Oils, 9 Vivian Avenue, Hendon Central, London NW4 3UT.

Aromatherapy Blends and Remedies by Franzesca Watson. Over 800 essential-oil recipes for everyday use.

Published by Thorsons
ISBN 0 7225 3222 9

Aromatherapy – A Nurses Guide for Women by Ann Percival. Not at all complicated. An easy read but with more technical and medical data for health professionals as well as lay readers.
Published by Amberwood
ISBN 1 899308 12 1
From health stores and bookshops. In case of difficulty, call Amberwood Publishing Limited on 01483 570821.

Aromatherapy – A Guide for Home Use by Christine Westwood. Just as the title says.
Published by Amberwood
ISBN 0 951 77230 9
From health stores and bookshops. In case of difficulty, call Amberwood Publishing Limited on 01483 570821

What Doctors Don't Tell You
Proof! and
The WDDTY Guide to Environmental Hazards.
For subscription information, send a large s.a.e. to: Wallace Press, 4 Wallace Road, London N1 2PG

The Inside Story. Specialist information for those with food allergies in the form of a regular mazine with recipes.
Published by Berrydale Publishers, Berrydale House, 5 Lawn Road, London NW3 2SX. Send an s.a.e. for details.

SOURCES OF REFERENCE

Colbin, A. 'Food and the Law of Opposites – Acid and Alkaline.' *Food and Healing* 73–80.

Hay, W.H. *Health Via Food*. The Sun-Diet Foundation, 1934.

Shelton, H.M. *Food Combining Made Easy*, 1951.

Tuormaa, T. 'Pesticides – The poisons all around us'. *What Doctors Don't Tell You*, June 1995, 6[3]:1–3.

'Updates': 'Sheep Pesticides: nerve disorders.' *What Doctors Don't Tell You*, July 1995, 6[4]:4.

Smith, Bob L. 'Organic foods vs supermarket foods: element levels.' *Journal of Applied Nutrition*, 1993, 45[1]:35–39.

'Harmful bacteria now on fresh produce: Report.' *Tufts University Diet & Nutrition Letter*, January 1997, 14[11]:1–2.

'Passive smoking can damage your health! Breathing other people's smoke: The effects of passive smoking.' Health Education Authority leaflet.

Zondervan, K.T et al. 'Do dietary and supplementary intakes of antioxidants differ with smoking status?' *International Journal of Epidemiology*, 1996, 25[1]:70–79.

Raloff J. 'The Gender Benders.' *Science News*, January 1994.

'Chemicals in home cleaning products.' *Townsend Letter for Doctors*, November 1994, 1272–74.

'Updates': 'Dioxin found in animal fats.' *What Doctors Don't Tell You*, November 1994:5[8]:5.

'Motorists warned of petrol health risk.' Press information released by The Associated Octel Company Limited, 4 November 1993.

Tierno, P.M, Hanna, B.A. 'Propensity of tampons and barrier contraceptives to amplify *Staphylococcus aureus* Toxic Shock Syndrome Toxin-1.' *Infectious Diseases in Obstetrics & Gynecology* 1994, 2:140–45.

'Sanitary Products.' *What Doctors Don't Tell You*, 1995, 6[7]:10–11.

Guyton, A.C. *Textbook of Medical Physiology*, Eighth edition, 1991, 726–28. Digestion and absorption in the gastrointestinal tract. Explanation of the different digestive processes of starch and protein.

Harvey, G. *The Killing of the Countryside*. Jonathan Cape.

'Toothpaste may cause periodontitis.' Letters to the Editor. *What Doctors Don't Tell You*, April 1997, 8[1]:5.

Behan, P. 'Chronic Fatigue Syndrome as a delayed reaction to chronic low-dose organophosphate exposure.' *Journal of Nutritional and Environmental Medicine*, 1996, 6:341–50.

'Pesticides.' RSPB magazine *Birds*, Summer 1997, 59.

'Another Silent Spring' (Television documentary). BBC2, Wednesday, 7 May 1997.

Personal discussions with Dr M.M. Verheyen on the health benefits of fasting and detoxification, and on liver function and digestive disorders. Teufen, Switzerland, August 1996.

'Special Report: Fuelling the carbohydrate weight gain facility.' *Tufts University Diet & Nutrition Letter*, 1995, 13[3]:4–6.

'Countryfile report.' BBC1, Sunday, 25 June 1997.

Page, Christine R. *Frontiers of Health*. C.W. Daniel. 'Liver disease/Gallstones' 163–4.

Dethlefsen, T. & Dahlke, R. *The Healing Power of Illness*, 138–42. Element. 'Digestion: The Liver/The Gallbladder.'

Tierra, M. 'Healing the liver, healing the body.' *International Journal of Alternative and Complementary Medicine*, February 1997, 23–25.

Leung, A. *The Encyclopedia of Common Natural Ingredients Used in Food, Drugs and Cosmetics*. John Wiley & Sons. [Unnumbered photocopied pages provided to me by the library service.]

Mills, S. *The Complete Guide to Modern Herbalism*. Thorsons. Cholagogue (62) Dandelion root (75).

Bunney, S. (ed.) *The Illustrated Encyclopedia of Herbs: Their Medicinal and Culinary Uses*. Aura Books.

Jensen, B., Bell, A. *Tissue Cleansing Through Bowel Management*. Bernard Jensen, 1981.

'Report gives excess toothpaste the brush-off.' *Tufts University Diet and Nutrition Letter*, 1996, 13[12]:1.

Reader Information

❧

The information that Kathryn includes in her books, feature articles and lectures has been accumulated from her own personal research, training and experience which, from the feedback she has received, would appear to have helped many people. However, it is important that the reader understands that these guidelines are not intended to be prescriptive, nor are they an attempt to diagnose or treat any specific condition.

Recommendations contained within the text are based on Kathryn's personal and clinical experience. Her views are completely independent. She is not employed by any pharmaceutical company, supplement supplier or food producer.

If you are concerned in any way about your health, Kathryn recommends that you visit your own doctor or hospital consultant without delay. She also suggests that you keep your medical adviser informed of any dietary changes and of any supplement programmes you intend to follow. Obtain as many details about your condition as possible, asking plenty of questions about any medicines which may be prescribed to you. Do not stop taking any currently prescribed medication without first talking with your general practitioner.

In the meantime, follow a varied and sensible diet that contains plenty of fresh unprocessed wholefoods, daily fresh fruits and vegetables, and filtered or bottled water. Take regular exercise and avoid cigarette smoke.

Kathryn regrets that, due to the cost and time involved in dealing with her already overloaded mailbag, she can no longer reply individually to letters nor is she able to comment on specific case histories. She is, however, always delighted to hear from readers and promises to read every letter.

A man was lost in the desert.

Later, when describing his ordeal to his friends, he told, how in sheer despair, he had knelt down and cried out for God to help him.

'And did God answer your prayer?' he was asked.

'Heavens no! But it was all right, thank goodness. A nomad appeared and showed me the way!'

Index

~